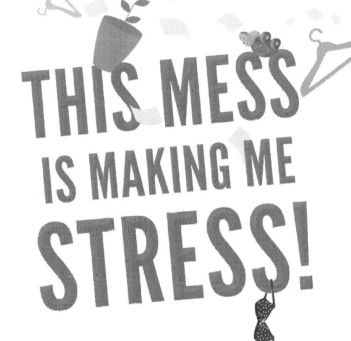

THIS MESS
IS MAKING ME
STRESS!

HOW TO
ORGANIZE YOUR HOME
AND FIND PEACE

DONNA BARWALD

- represents unrealized dreams
- makes you feel inadequate or ashamed
- you think was meaningful to someone else
- you have two of them because you forgot you already had one
- you have three of them because you couldn't find the first two

By now, everyone knows how to declutter by sorting stuff into piles: keep, donate, sell, and trash. But our stuff is imbued with emotions, not all of them positive. When you look at your stuff, negative emotions derail you before you begin.

How can you decide anything when you're stressed and depressed? I will teach you a method that helps you, starting with small decisions and building up to tougher ones. The goal is to let go of the wrong stuff and begin a habit of daily organizing and maintaining what's left.

Letting go of the wrong stuff makes space for the right stuff to surround you: improved self-esteem, confidence, a calmer mind, a better energy flow – as well as rooms that function better and a home that brings you joy.

I've seen it work, and it will work for you too! Using the advice in this book will improve your mood, help you feel better about yourself, and give you the strength and the tools you need to start and keep organizing. Your home will be neatly arranged, but more than that, you will be transformed. Instead of your home driving you crazy, you will find peace (and your stuff, too!).

PART 1

Assessing Your Stress

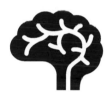

Chapter 1

Stressed and Depressed

Twenty years ago, I started a professional organizing business called Neatly Arranged. My twin sister jokingly calls it Nearly Deranged because when we were growing up, our disorganized home drove me so crazy that I would wake up early in the morning before the rest of my family and rearrange the kitchen. I did not score points with them, but it was a way I could control my environment.

Over the years, I have gained much insight into the help people need to turn their living and working spaces, which are causing stress, into organized surroundings that give them peace. The help isn't just practical; it's emotional too. Listening, understanding, and working through your mental roadblocks are just as crucial as getting suitable containers and labeling. My goal is to improve your quality of life, not just make your home look better. Anyone can take "before and after" pictures of an organized room. I'm more interested in the "before and after" of your state of mind.

Psychological Implications of Clutter

I have a wonderful friend Monica who is an artist and therapist. She helped me put together a program a few years back called "Creating Peace by Creating Space," where we discussed the psychological implications of clutter and the importance of organizing for mental health. Monica started the workshop with the following exercise, which helps you understand how clutter affects you.

ASK YOURSELF...

1. Where do you feel peaceful?

- What is it about that space that helps you feel that way?
- What does it look like?
- Where are you in the space?
- What is the light like?
- What are the textures of the space and the colors?
- What are the things in that space, and how do you see them?

2. Where do you feel stressed?

- What is it about that space that makes you feel that way?
- What does it look like?
- What is the lighting like?
- How much room do you have to move?
- Are you alone or with others?
- What are the things in that space, and how do you see them?

3. How does your environment, the space you spend the most time in, affect your well-being?

If you are like most people, the places where you feel stressed are cluttered. That isn't to say that your environment needs to be minimalist to be peaceful. Peace comes from carefully curating your environment, so it is filled with things you love rather than things that randomly land there and arranging it in a harmonious way that leaves enough space for energy to flow.

During the COVID-19 pandemic and the lockdown in Los Angeles, which closed schools and many businesses for more than a year, my organizing business (like many other businesses) disappeared because people couldn't invite me into their homes. How ironic since people suddenly had plenty of time and opportunity to organize. Some people took the opportunity to declutter their closets and get rid of old clothes and toys. Some cleaned up the backyard or tried to tackle the dreaded garage. Being at home forced people to look at what was there. But for many, looking at what was there was depressing, and it was easier physically and emotionally just to shut the door and watch Netflix. Sound familiar?

How Clutter Affects Us

During our workshop, Monica shared that not only is she affected by clutter, but she is also affected by anything being in the wrong place where it doesn't belong. Her family does not experience the environment the same way. She calls them "collectors," and they leave "trails." To escape the anxiety of clutter, she created her own retreat which started as a corner of the living room in which to have coffee in peace and now has become a full-blown artist studio built in her backyard. What is it about clutter that gives us anxiety and makes us stressed?

Clutter makes us anxious because the piles seem never-ending. Relaxing is more difficult because it signals to our brains that our work is never done. I often feel guilty when I want to watch something or work on my hobbies because there is so much to do.

Clutter pulls focus and reduces productivity. It draws our attention away from what our focus should be because our brain needs to work overtime to respond to excessive, unnecessary stimuli. Clutter invades the space we need to dream, create, and problem-solve.

Clutter affects our relationships. It impedes our ability to find things quickly, so we arrive late, miss deadlines, and inconvenience people. We tend to apologize a lot. We feel ashamed because we think we should be more organized. We have this idea in our head that our self-worth depends on the tidiness of our home, so we feel "less than."

Clutter hurts our social life. Our home should be a place to feel pride. Instead, we are reluctant to invite people over because we don't want people to judge us by our clutter, and we are embarrassed when people drop by.

Clutter leads to unhealthy eating. Research at Cornell University showed that people would eat more cookies and snacks if the environment in which they're offered a choice of foods is chaotic, and they're led to feel stressed.[1] When the experimental kitchen in which participants were tested was disorganized and messy, and they were put in a low self-control mindset, students in the lab ate twice as many cookies as those in a standard, non-chaotic kitchen. In other words, when you feel out of control, you'll reach more for the sweets in a cluttered setting.

Clutter makes it harder to read people's feelings. In examining the impact of clutter on perceptions of scenes in movies, researchers in a 2016 study at Cornell University found that when the background of a scene is highly cluttered, viewers find it more challenging to interpret the emotional expressions on the faces of the characters.[2] Applied to daily life, you'll be less accurate in figuring out how others feel when you see them amidst a clutter-filled room. I imagine that's why it's easier to "read the room" in a conference room or lecture hall, and people who have trouble with social cues do better in a less crowded and uncluttered environment.

Clutter contributes to memory problems. I'm not just talking about losing your keys because they're hidden under a pile of papers. University of Toronto's Lynn Hasher's research suggests that mental clutter is a leading cause of age-related memory loss. The visual distraction of clutter increases cognitive overload and can reduce working memory.[3]

I was a computer teacher, so think of it this way: Your brain is like a computer. If too many tabs open simultaneously (visual clutter), your processor will run slower. Plus, all those extraneous tabs take up storage space, so there is less space to move around and access the necessary files you have stored.

Your Brain on Clutter

Picture this:

You are home, and instead of feeling safe and peaceful, your senses are working overtime, taking in a mess. The amygdala (the part of your brain that processes emotion) perceives a stressor (clutter). It signals the hypothalamus to stimulate the sympathetic nervous system, which prepares the body to respond to the threat. The adrenal glands release stress hormones like adrenaline and cortisol into the bloodstream, forcing you to stay tense and alert and causing the reaction to Fight, Flight, or Freeze.

- **Fight** - you "tackle" the clutter, or you get angry and argue with the people making the mess
- **Flight** - you shut the door, avoid the job, and distract yourself with something else
- **Freeze** - you are paralyzed and overwhelmed - you don't know how to start, so you take a nap, and nothing gets done.

Stress Changes Your Brain

Imagine being in a chronically cluttered environment and constantly in that tense, high-alert state. There has been a lot of research into the harmful effects of stress on your brain. As if you weren't stressed enough before, check this out:

- **Stress Changes Brain Structure.** It upsets the balance between gray and white matter, which can result in long-term changes to brain structures and function.
- **Stress Kills Brain Cells.** It produces high cortisol levels, killing new neurons in the hippocampus – an area associated with learning, memory, and emotion and where new brain cells are formed.[4]
- **Stress Shrinks the Brain.** It reduces grey matter in the prefrontal cortex – the part of the brain associated with memory and emotional regulation.[5]
- **Stress Increases the Risk of Mental Illness.** People who undergo prolonged periods of stress are more prone to suffer from mood and anxiety disorders later in life because of long-term changes to the brain.

Key Takeaway

Mess causes stress which adversely affects your physical and mental health. An ongoing practice of organizing is just as important as meditation, exercise, and diet for your overall well-being.

Chapter 2

Listen to Your Clutter

The Clutter Feedback Loop

The psychological effects of clutter act as a feedback loop. A feedback loop occurs when the cause (input) produces an effect (output) which then becomes the cause, endlessly trapping us in a loop.

We build our clutter around a psychological component:

- uncontrolled consumer impulses
- emotional sentiment
- memories of the past
- fear of a future need
- guilt or obligation
- hope for a change in the future

Then the clutter itself results in adverse psychological effects: stress, feelings of shame or inadequacy, poor attention span, and negative behaviors (like unhealthy eating). Then those adverse psychological effects encourage us to buy more items that comfort us or cling tighter to the ones we currently have.

What is Your Clutter Saying?

If your clutter is an excess of unused items, it could be because:

- you use "retail therapy" to feel better ("I deserve new shoes.")
- you have a fear of the future ("You never know when you might need this.")
- you wish you were something you're not ("I'm going to learn to play guitar.")

- you long for the day when you have time ("I'll need these scrapbook supplies.")

If your clutter is largely memorabilia from your past, then:

- you may have trouble letting things go or forgiving (old correspondence)
- you feel like your best days are behind you (trophies)
- you feel an obligation to document your history

If your clutter is other people's things, it could be:

- you don't want to lose your memories of them
- you feel obligated to keep things, or they will get mad
- you feel guilty for getting rid of something meaningful to someone
- you hope they will come back for it someday

If you have a lot of unfinished projects, it could mean:

- you are a perfectionist - you can't finish it because it will never be good enough; it serves as a reminder of your failure to do something you set out to do
- you feel obligated to do things, so you start a project and then abandon it
- you have bursts of energy or inspiration before reality hits, and you lose hope or motivation

Key Takeaway

Understanding why you accumulate and keep things will explain your difficulty in decluttering and organizing. Take a minute to identify the psychological source of your clutter.

Chapter 3

You Might Be Neurodivergent

OCD or Just Neat?

We throw around the term "OCD" a lot these days, often laughing it off as a quirk of someone who likes things extremely neat. Just because they spend a lot of time keeping their home clean and organized doesn't mean they have OCD (obsessive-compulsive disorder)! They could merely enjoy the flow of energy an organized home provides.

The difference is OCD causes extreme anxiety and involves obsessions and compulsions that interfere with daily life. One obsession could be keeping everything overly organized. They don't just like everything neat and orderly; they feel compelled to keep it that way and suffer great distress if they don't. Believe it or not, in some cases, OCD could look like the polar opposite of how we usually think. It could be an extremely cluttered home because hoarding is a type of OCD. A mental health professional must diagnose OCD and its associated disorders.

You're Not a Hoarder!

25% of people with OCD also have compulsive hoarding. Compulsive hoarding is also considered a feature of obsessive-compulsive personality disorder (OCPD) and may develop with other mental illnesses. But just because you have a lot of stuff and find it challenging to get rid of things doesn't necessarily mean you're a hoarder.

According to the American Psychiatric Association (2013), specific symptoms for a hoarding disorder diagnosis include:

- Persistent difficulty discarding or parting with possessions, regardless of their actual value.
- This difficulty is due to a perceived need to save the items and to the distress associated with discarding them.
- The difficulty discarding possessions results in the accumulation of possessions that congest and clutter active living areas and substantially compromises their intended use. If living areas are uncluttered, it is only because of the interventions of third parties (e.g., family members, cleaners, or the authorities.)
- The hoarding causes clinically significant distress or impairment in social, occupational, or other important areas of functioning (including maintaining a safe environment safe for oneself or others.)

Unless your home is a fire hazard and every room is so cluttered that you can't move around and resist doing anything about it, you are not a hoarder. Hoarding disorder is such a debilitating condition that I don't think you would have the presence of mind to read this book if you were.

If you wish to declutter, and your physical health or ability to focus prevents you from doing so, you are not a hoarder. You may, however, be neurodivergent.

Neurodivergence is a Difference

Neurodivergent describes a person whose brain processes the world differently than most people. Autism, Attention Deficit Hyperactivity Disorder (ADHD), OCD, Tourette Syndrome, dyslexia, and other learning differences fall under the category of neurodivergent.

Research is ongoing into the genetic and environmental causes of neurodivergence, and it tends to run in families. It is possible to become neurodiverse due to a physical or emotional injury or trauma. Still, in most cases, neurodivergence is something you are born with, like giftedness or left-handedness.

When Your Executive Function Isn't Functional

Neurodiverse people often have challenges with Executive Function—the set of skills that help someone plan and achieve a goal:

- Flexible thinking
- Initiating
- Planning
- Prioritization
- Self-monitoring
- Self-control
- Working memory
- Time management
- Organization

As it is with artistic talent or athletic ability, some people are born with strong executive function skills. If that is not your gift, there are strategies you can learn, and many people hire an executive function coach to help.

There's an App for That

Search in Google Play or Apple App Store for executive function, time management, scheduling, planning, or organizing. You will find dozens of apps and games made specifically to help with executive function skills.

Now You Know

So, if you have wondered why you seem to struggle so much with organizing when it appears to come easy to others, now you know.

Strong negative emotions often stop us in our tracks. You hit the wall as soon as you begin. Recognizing and accepting what you truly feel when overwhelmed will help you get through it. So, take a moment to focus on your emotions. Do any of these resonate with you?

- Despair: I tried, but it's hopeless!
- Anger: I can't get anyone to cooperate!
- Sadness: I can't right now; I'm grieving.
- Anxiety: I'm afraid I'll regret the decision.
- Loneliness: I want a friend to help me.
- Frustration: I can't do this until I do that.
- Depression: I don't have the energy.

You've heard, "feel the fear and do it anyway." I suggest you feel your emotion, acknowledge it, and organize anyway. Your feelings don't have to stop you – just be creative and think of ways to use them while you organize.

You can do small actions that will produce noticeable results and put you in control. Even a hint of progress brings hope, and hope will keep you going.

When you feel despair:

- Make your bed.
- Organize office supplies.
- Plan to transform a space into a different use.

When you feel angry:

- Rip up junk mail.
- Tear pages out of spiral notebooks.
- Throw broken things into the trash.

When you feel sad:

- Sort pillows and blankets.
- Organize tissues and toilet paper.
- Neatly arrange your teas.

When you feel anxious:

- Get online appraisals for things you think are valuable.
- Organize the refrigerator.
- Throw out burnt or scratched pots.

When you feel lonely:

- Call a friend while you clean.
- Tidy the living room.
- Invite guests, so you have more motivation.

When you feel frustrated:

- Shred papers.
- Organize batteries.
- Manage power cords.

When you are depressed:

- Label the remotes.
- Declutter the coffee table.
- Match socks.

These activities meet you where you are emotionally and, in some cases, physically (on the couch when you are depressed, in bed when you're sad). In general, they don't take a lot of decision-making, so they're not as taxing on your brain. What other activities can you come up with?

Declutter Regret

I have a friend whose idea of decluttering is "Take no prisoners!" She has no problem giving away things and eagerly commands others to do the same. That's fine for her because she lives where it is easy to buy anything she may need to replace, and she has the money to do it. She is also in the business of buying and selling, so she has experience in knowing what things are worth. Not everyone has that opportunity or experience.

Declutter regret is the leading reason that prevents people from decluttering. It is the fear of being foolish for giving away something valuable or the anxiety from thinking they won't have the means or the ability to rebuy something if needed.

I have had clients reluctantly decide to get rid of something and later retrieve it from the trash bin or the donation center because they second-guess themselves. Being afraid to make a mistake paralyzes people with indecision, and I often have to reassure them that they are making a good decision when they finally do.

Take Time to Research

To overcome the anxiety, I believe the more information you have, the more confident you can be in your decisions. Learning more about something you feel you need to keep can ease your mind and make it easier to decide the fate of a possession.

Take the time to look up the price or availability of something you think you might need to buy again. If you're keeping something you don't need or like just because you think it's worth something, get an online appraisal of items you think may be valuable and see at what price similar items sold. Make sure it's worth your time and money to store it and sell it later. At the end of the book, there are resources for appraising and selling online.

Depression is Both Cause and Effect

Depression is a cause keeping you from organizing and an effect of your home needing organizing. People with depression don't have the energy to do much, and organizing, with its physical and mental demands, is the last thing any depressed person wants to do. "I don't have the strength for this right now" means your ability to problem-solve and make decisions are impaired.

Depression makes decision-making difficult, if not impossible, and ambiguity is not conducive to decluttering. With no energy to get off the couch and no bandwidth to make decisions, you let things go, making you even more depressed!

Take a Shower

So, what can you do besides therapy and medication (which I strongly recommend)? First, take a shower. The negative ions from running water will give you a little boost, and while you're in the shower, go through the bottles of shampoo, conditioner, body wash, and shaving cream -- anything empty you can throw out? Can you group them so they look nicer? That's a start.

When you pick out a towel, can you pull out the ragged ones and rip them up for rags? That's progress! If that's all you have energy for today, fine.

If you still have energy and time, do a little more while in the bathroom. Even If five minutes is all you can handle, you're making progress, and soon you will be strong enough to do more.

Key Takeaway

Our belongings are infused with emotions, and strong negative emotions stop us from organizing. By acknowledging these feelings, you can work through them and take specific actions to continue organizing.

Chapter 5

Eating a Plum

Sometimes I feel sorry for myself because everyone else has somewhere to go, and here I am, home alone, with a house to clean and organize but no desire to do any of it. It reminds me of being a kid and not getting to go out with my friends because I have to stay home and clean my room. It feels like punishment, like being grounded.

Organizing can be lonely, but it doesn't have to be. It doesn't have to feel like punishment if you make it into a social opportunity. My friends and I call it *"Eating a Plum."*

Years ago, my friend struggled to put in her contact lenses. She couldn't do it alone, so she asked her dad to come over and help her. He did, and he kept helping her until she could do it alone one day. Then she just needed her dad for moral support. He would come over, sit there while she put on her contacts, and eat a plum.

These days, when we need someone to keep us company while we do something we find difficult, we ask them to come over and eat a plum. Having a friend over makes the task less lonely and more fun.

Friends and Neighbors are Necessary

In past generations, women cooked and cleaned and raised kids together, and it helped alleviate the loneliness of staying home. Neighbors were more than just people you saw when you got in and out of your car; they helped each other.

Now I'm not saying you should ask your neighbor to help organize your garage (that's what spouses are for), but you can ask a friend to come over while you tackle the kid's room, clean out the pantry, or turn a junk room into a guest room. Then be there for them when they need you to eat a plum.

Key Takeaway

Ask a friend to keep you company while you organize to make the work more enjoyable.

Chapter 6

Ten Things First

It's common to feel frustrated because you don't have what you need to tackle the job, don't have the time to complete the task, have tried before without success, or hit an obstacle you don't know how to overcome. It's the phenomenon of "Ten Things First."

Think about what you might go through organizing a home office:

1. I can't file the papers because the file drawers are too full.
2. I can't make room in the filing cabinet until I know what I can throw out.
3. I have to see if I have digital copies saved on the old computer.
4. I can't look at the old computer because it doesn't work.
5. I need to transfer the information on the hard drive to my new computer.
6. I can't do that myself, so I need the Geek Squad.
7. I don't want to wait in line, so I must make an appointment.
8. I have to look at my calendar first.
9. I don't want to make two trips, so I have to think about what else I need.
10. I know the printer needs ink, but I need to see which one.

See? You must do ten things before you can even file, let alone accomplish your goal of organizing the office!

But even if you hit a roadblock, you can keep moving forward by diverting your attention to other spaces or organizing tasks: setting reminders, scheduling appointments, making calls, shopping online, listing things to donate and sell, and sorting papers, even if you can't file them yet.

Key Takeaway

People often get frustrated and stop organizing because they hit a roadblock that delays their progress. Even if that happens, there is always something you can do to keep the momentum of organizing: sorting, planning, shopping, scheduling, and the like.

Chapter 7

The Wrong Stuff

With all those emotions going on, it's no wonder why organizing is difficult. It would be much easier if everything you saw or touched didn't bring up such negative feelings or make you feel bad about yourself. It would be a pleasure if you only organize things that bring you joy.

Think about your holiday decorations. Can you have too many decorations? Not if they are put away in tubs on shelves, and you can get to them when the holiday comes. Organizing your decorations is work, but it's pleasant, and unless you've had a recent loss, I'm pretty sure strong emotions don't prevent you from doing it. (Frustration with the tangle of lights doesn't count.)

Now think about any collection you've ever had. Organizing a collection Is enjoyable because you can look at what you have and surround yourself with things you love that bring up happy memories. Remember Carrie Bradshaw's room-sized closet from *Sex and the City*? The designer clothes, hats, shoes, and accessories were all beautiful, they all fit, and they all brought happy memories. Everything was neatly arranged, and it was nirvana every time she opened that closet.

It was a lot of stuff, but it wasn't too much. It was the right stuff because It made her happy; she had room to store everything neatly without visual clutter, and she could easily see and access it.

The problem isn't that you have *too much* stuff. The problem is that the *wrong* stuff surrounds you, and it's not good for your mental health.

Painful Stuff

One of my very first clients had files upon files in file drawers. I could tell right away he didn't need half those papers. Some were from a business he'd lost years ago due to a partner's unfair business practices. Some were my client's bitter divorce and custody arrangements, even though the kids were now grown and flown. These chapters of his life still made him furious, yet he kept these things around.

When your past holds hurt and anger, you want to leave it and move forward. No one wants to be reminded of it. Even looking at a document is painful, so *it* sits. In this client's case, he never threw anything out -- good, bad, or indifferent -- and forgot that he had it. He didn't need the business stuff for taxes, and even if he ever needed the divorce decree again, he didn't have to keep all the pleadings and filings and the back-and-forth of who was paying for the kids' braces. But even when I brought it up, why couldn't he throw it away?

You're Not the President

Some of us feel our lives must be documented and stored like a presidential library, as if a biographer will need all this stuff one day so they can get all the details right. We need evidence of every feeling we've ever had, whether positive feelings like joy, love, accomplishment, and success, or negative feelings like anger, hurt, loss, and rejection.

That's why getting rid of cards, gifts, souvenirs, pictures, report cards, test scores, acceptance letters, trophies, and awards is so hard. You want to memorialize those happy moments. Yet divorce papers, letters from lost loves, rejection letters, statements from bad investments, and former friends' belongings are unhappy memories. No one wants to feel those negative feelings when we uncover the past, so it's no wonder we can't bring ourselves to organize. Happy memories are the right stuff; unhappy memories are the wrong stuff.

Critical Stuff

Another kind of wrong stuff is things that make you feel bad about yourself, that feed into that critical voice that says you're foolish, inadequate, gullible, not good enough. While it makes sense to hold onto things of value, people also hold onto things that make them feel foolish for spending money on them.

I had a client who still beats herself up for paying more than twice what she should have for a beautiful piece of art she has to pass to go to the front door. Even though she bought it years ago, it makes her wince whenever she passes it. I understand wanting to get pleasure out of something you paid dearly for, but if it's going to make you feel bad multiple times a day, is it worth it? That's why it's the wrong stuff.

I am guilty of it too. The last time I looked through my memory box, I saw rejection letters from when I applied for a government grant and a graduate program right out of college. Why did I keep them? To remind me 40 years later how foolish and unqualified I was to apply at that time? Time to let them go.

It is much easier to deal with other wrong stuff because you must build up to going through the stuff laden with negative emotions.

Broken Stuff

It's hard to understand why people keep a broken thing when they've replaced it with a new one, especially if seeing the broken item makes them angry all over again. Unless it is sentimental and goes into the memory box, you will feel better with it gone, and I don't just mean out of sight. If it's not usable, it clutters your home with the wrong stuff.

If it doesn't fit in the garbage, put it on the curb or call for a bulky item pickup. Call a hauling service if you can't get it to the curb or need it gone sooner. The same thing goes for things that are torn, ripped, stained, frayed, worn out, or faded -- if you already have a better one, there's no use in keeping it unless you need a rag, in which case, put it with the rags instead of cluttering up the nice closet.

Same Stuff

If something is not broken, but you've already replaced it, clearly you like the new one better. So why keep the old one?

Many people have similar things in the same category for different occasions, like vases, tablecloths, and glassware. When you put similar things together, it's easy to pick favorites to keep.

People often have more than one of the same or similar things because they've forgotten they had one or couldn't find it when needed. Unless there are legitimate reasons to keep more than one or two of the same thing (like reading glasses or office supplies), multiple items take up precious storage space for no reason, because you usually end up using the same one or two.

Obsolete Stuff

I can get into trouble with this one because if I say, "Why are you keeping the PlayStation no one is using?", my friend's husband will show me how much his original Atari is worth. Obsolete electronics may be worth something someday, but their potential value has to be measured against whether you have room to keep the things and whether you can do what it takes to sell them later.

It's hard to tell if your model is worth saving, but unless it was rare when it was new, the market would likely be flooded with them. If you are keeping something only because you think it might be worth something, see if it is! If you decide to keep it, store it well and label it so others won't inadvertently throw it away as junk.

Someone Else's Stuff

I was fortunate enough to have my great-grandmother with me until I was almost out of college and inherited some of her furnishings for my first apartment when she passed. Over the years, those things went back and forth between me, my grandmother, my mom, and my sisters. I now have a few of my favorite pieces back. Not because they were Nana's, but because I love them. I could have had many more, but just a few beautiful things were enough for me.

Grandma's Treasure

I knew someone with a very ugly tchotchke (knick-knack) that they only kept because they remembered seeing it in their grandmother's house and thought it meant a lot to her.

My friend's mother came over one day, saw it, and asked with surprise, "Why do you have this ugly thing?" "Because it was one of Grandma's treasures," my friend answered. Her mom laughed. "Aunt Betty gave her that. Your grandma hated it and only displayed it to be nice when Aunt Betty came over." My friend realized they had only been at their grandmother's house when Aunt Betty was there!

The story's moral is that just because it was Grandma's doesn't mean she had a special attachment. So, if you are keeping things you don't love just because you think they meant something to someone you love, don't. That's the wrong stuff. Feel free to pass it on.

Borrowed and Forgotten Stuff

Whenever I help my daughter go through her room, she inevitably finds clothes and things she borrowed from a friend that she neglected to return. This kind of wrong stuff hangs around, cluttering the place until you go out of your way to return it.

Put a bag of things you must return by the front door or in your car. This advice also goes for textbooks and library books, for which you'll pay a fine. Then it will be the wrong stuff because it will make you angry with yourself every time you see it.

Clear Your Conscience

If you have no idea who it belongs to or have no way to get it to them -- and you don't want it yourself -- donate it. That includes Blockbuster tapes, Netflix DVDs, and library books for which you've already paid a late fee. If evidence of a past mistake still makes you feel guilty or ashamed, clear your conscience and eliminate it. You don't need Jiminy Cricket hanging around, making you feel bad for something you forgot to do a long time ago.

In addition, if you still have something left behind by someone you broke up with or who did you wrong, letting go is long overdue. If something brings up strong negative emotions every time you look at it, it's not worth affecting your mental health.

Stuff in Storage Units

Anything sitting in a paid storage unit for more than seven years is the wrong stuff for most people. You don't need to keep tax documents for more than seven years. Seven years after a loss, you have likely passed through the stages of grief and can look at things again. If you've needed to use something in the last seven years, it probably stayed in your home. Very few people use storage units to bring things back and forth.

Unless you have a storage unit full of priceless memories or a collection of value like art, baseball cards, or a classic car, I can't imagine paying at least $100 a month for seven years for storage. Seven years at that price is $8,400! Even if it's an antique piece of furniture, is it worth more than $8,400?

Is It Good for Me or Not?

Are you with me so far? If I say you have too much stuff, you might get defensive and want to hold on to everything. You may agree and feel ashamed, inadequate, or both, and still be unable to pare down. "Too much" brings up strong emotions, and intense emotions are the most significant barrier to organizing.

Looking through the lens of "is it good for my mental, spiritual, and physical well-being," diffuses the defensiveness and the need to keep the wrong stuff. Your job is to be a decluttering detective and root out the wrong stuff as the prime targets to sell, give away, or trash.

Key Takeaway

Anything that doesn't benefit you mentally, spiritually, or physically is the wrong stuff and the prime target of your decluttering.

PART 2

Finding Peace by Creating Space

Chapter 8

Room to Breathe

When I first meet a client, I walk around their home with them and ask what happens in each room. I hear things like:

- "This is the dining room, but we always eat in the kitchen, so we never use it."
- "This used to be my office, but it's turned into a junk room."
- "They use this computer to do homework, but I can't supervise here."
- "I wanted to do yoga and work out here, but it's too dark and depressing."
- "This used to be a guest room until the kids took it over with their video games."
- "I would use this as a sewing room if there were more room and storage."

This Isn't Working for Me

There's always a reason why a room doesn't seem to function as you intend or is a challenge to keep organized.

- It may need to be rearranged for better flow.
- It needs additional storage space.
- The environment needs improvement with better light or temperature control, more outlets, or wi-fi connectivity.
- There are things in there that need to find another home.
- The room is better suited to be used for something else altogether.

Sometimes a room doesn't work because so many negative feelings arise every time you pass by or go in that you can't even stand to be in there. You may be:

- Sad that your kid has moved out of their bedroom or annoyed that they left everything for you to pack.
- Aggravated that you can't get to what you need in the garage because no one will help you.
- Conflicted because the antique furniture from Grandma is cluttering the family room, but you can't get rid of it.
- Resentful because you gave up the lease on your office space, and now your home office is cluttered with that furniture.
- Frustrated that the kitchen is still a mess, and you can't decide which flooring and backsplash to put in.

These are examples I've encountered over the years. All those negative feelings keep you stuck and unable to enjoy your home. So, what can you do?

You'll See it When You Believe It

Self-help guru Wayne Dyer wrote a motivational book that turns the old expression "I'll believe it when I see it" on its head. "You'll see it when you believe it" encourages us to dream. If all you can see is what's wrong, it makes it hard to see the possibilities of what could be right. When all you see is clutter, you get demoralized because you don't have the energy or right mind frame to deal with it. To counteract that, I'm asking you to dream!

Dream, Dream, Dream

Dream about the lifestyle you want, and then apply it to the home you have.

If you have kids, it might be:

- "I want to be able to watch my kids doing homework, and I don't want to hear their video games."
- "I want to be cozy on my couch watching Disney+ with the kids."
- "I want my kids to have a play area separate from their bedroom, so I'm not stepping on Legos when I put them to bed, and have it be easy for them to put away their toys."
- "It would be lovely if I could retreat with my husband upstairs and have snacks and beverages right there like a hotel without going down to the kitchen and getting bombarded with kids needing me."

If you want more work/life balance:

- "I want to work from home on a laptop in a light, airy room with a view."
- "I want to be able to do yoga and Pilates on a nice floor and watch TV while I'm on the elliptical."
- "I want to be able to entertain friends on a moment's notice and have big family dinners on holidays."
- "It would be great to have a space to be creative, with my Cricut and art supplies stored in a way I can easily access them."

If you want to make life easier, it could be:

- "I want to know exactly where good batteries and scissors are when I need them and space to wrap presents without my family seeing."

- "I like to buy huge packages from Costco to save money, but I don't want to go out to the garage when I need a roll of paper towels."
- "I would like it to be easy, not a hassle, getting my kids out to school with the signed papers, sports equipment, backpacks, and jackets they need."

Maybe This Could Work

Now, look around your home and see what spaces could work for the things you want to do. It doesn't have to be a whole room.

- Is there a space with a view and great light to sit with your laptop and be productive?
- How about a play area with storage that can be cleaned up quickly?
- Or a guest room that can double as a video game room?
- Is there space to turn part of your bedroom into a sitting room near an outlet to plug in a mini-fridge?
- What about a floorspace close to a TV with room for exercise equipment?
- Maybe a dining room can double as a craft and wrapping room?
- Homework space near the kitchen so you can keep an eye on kids while you are figuring out schedules and making dinner?

Make it Manifest

When you designate a space for a specific activity and dream about how it will feel being in that space doing that activity, it helps you get past what's keeping you stuck and motivates you to do something to make it manifest. It's easier and more fun to clear out a room of a kid who is "grown and flown" when you can direct your energy towards a new venture, like a craft room where your creativity can flourish.

I know you're thinking, "But I can't do all that by myself!" You don't have to! That's what kids, partners, friends, handymen, organizers, and Eagle Scouts are for.

Once you have a dream and can get others to buy into your vision, it is much easier to ask for help. "Can you please help me create a craft room?" produces better results than "I need you to help me clean up and organize the back bedroom."

Zone In

Once you've decided the general purpose of a room, you will arrange (or rearrange) the room into zones that make sense for what you want to do there and make you feel good being there. Let's use the example of a family room where people spend time together.

➢ **Identify what you intend to do in this room.**

- watching TV
- playing video games
- making music
- exercising
- doing homework
- playing games
- doing arts and crafts
- opening presents under the tree
- dancing
- having sleepovers
- building a fort

➢ **Now decide what furniture and equipment you need to do those things.**

- couch
- coffee table
- TV stand for audio/visual equipment and media storage
- guitar and a piano,
- table with at least four chairs
- desk or table with a chair and a computer
- exercise equipment with a yoga mat and floor space
- storage for school supplies, arts and crafts supplies, board games, blankets, and pillows

➢ **Take the environment into consideration.**

- light
- acoustics
- temperature
- wi-fi connectivity
- location of walls, windows, doors
- Location of electrical outlets and phone/cable connectors
- HVAC registers and returns on the walls and ceiling
- existing storage: closets, cabinets, or shelves

These are generally the parameters of your layout. But if you have time and money, you can get an electrician to install new outlets or lighting, a cabinet maker to build extra storage, and a contractor to change anything else. Of course, it makes life easier and less expensive if you can arrange your space to maximize what you already have to work with.

Solving the Puzzle of Placement

Now comes the fun part. Where things go is not just a matter of where things fit.

Where you place everything is like solving a puzzle because not only does the piece need to go in the correct zone, but where it is placed has to meet the piece's requirements, AND it needs to fit.

For example:

- The TV needs to be on the wall where the outlets are, and the room needs to get dark enough to enjoy a movie in the daytime and not have glare.
- The couch and coffee table need to go across from the TV, but the couch cannot block the heat register and needs an outlet if it reclines.
- The piano needs a place with good acoustics and doesn't need electricity, but it cannot be near a heat source or a window if you want it to stay in tune.
- The turntable needs an outlet, and the vinyl records should be stored nearby, but they will warp if you play them too close to the fireplace.
- The computer needs to be near an outlet and have a wired internet connection or a strong wi-fi signal, in front of a window for natural light and across from a pleasant background to help you look good in video calls.
- The treadmill or elliptical needs to face the TV with floor space in between, with good light but not near the heat register.
- Storage to hold equipment for an activity needs to be near where the activity takes place.

Furniture with Storage

Look at the furniture you have that you can use to complete a zone. If you have a choice, always opt for pieces with storage.

- Can you use a trunk for a coffee table?
- An ottoman with storage for a seat?
- A table with plastic drawers underneath for a desk?
- A buffet or sideboard with drawers and cabinets as an audio/visual center?

Be creative and look at the whole house to find what you need. Re-orienting furniture can be a great solution. A shelf unit with cubbies can be used vertically like a bookcase or horizontally at kid height with baskets for storage.

Make Use of Wall Space

Consider using wall space for:

- Shelves and cubbies – Ikea has excellent solutions.
- Guitar hangers
- Speakers disguised as art
- Hooks for earphones or backpacks
- Magnetic whiteboard to store supplies in addition to writing on it
- Pegboard with accessories to store art, school, and office supplies

Creative Versatility

If you have a small space, you may want to use pieces that have double duty. For example, a piano bench can be used for extra storage or seating, and a trunk can be a coffee table and storage for extra sheets and blankets.

Anything on wheels or casters can be moved between zones as needed. You can add a tabletop accessory to a rolling cart to have storage for art supplies and a workspace. You can also use it as an end table, a dinner tray, or a desk to do homework on a laptop.

Organizing Is More Than Decluttering

The goal of organizing is to create a space that functions well and makes you feel calm and peaceful. You make a room work by designing a layout that makes sense for what you intend to do in that room, with furniture and storage that meets those requirements. When a room works, there is an ease of movement, and clutter has less opportunity to accumulate. There is a great energy flow, and the air feels lighter. You quite literally have room to breathe.

Key Takeaway

To organize a peaceful room that works, consider the environment and the activities you want to do there. Make creative use of versatile objects and wall space that can also serve as storage.

Chapter 9

Decisions, Decisions

When I was a kid, whenever I needed "space," I would lock myself up in the bathroom and organize the cabinet under the sink. I shared a bedroom with my twin sister, so the bathroom was the only place in the house where I could be by myself, and like the kitchen, the cabinet under the sink was one of the only things over which I had control.

I was tightly controlled by a father who had so many rules I had little opportunity to make decisions for myself. As a result, on the rare occasion when I dared to make my own decision, it was invariably the wrong one (according to my parents), and I often got punished for it.

I learned to fear making any decision at all. My decision-making muscles were weak, and I lost confidence in my ability. I couldn't even decide what to wear in the morning and needed approval for each outfit, so I didn't suffer the consequences of my wrong decision.

Fast forward to my college years when the big decision to move out was made for me – my dad kicked me out of the house! At 20 years old, I now had no choice but to make my own decisions – some of them not great, some of them the jury is still out, and some of them I'm lucky to be alive! But at least I had control.

Over the next 40 years, I built up those decision-making muscles. I moved at least 17 times. Every time you move, you have to think about everything you own because you don't want to waste money, time, and energy moving or storing it. So, it got easier to decide what to keep or let go.

Even though I still need help deciding what to wear sometimes, I can at least decide what to surround myself with and how to organize it all in a way that brings me peace.

Build Your Organizing Muscles

Like working out, organizing isn't something you do once; you do it for the rest of your life and build up to the heavy lifting. You can think of me as a personal trainer, and my goal is to help you build your organizing muscles so you can continue to organize.

We start with small, lightweight decisions where the consequences of making the wrong one are small, and then we add heavier decisions with more weight as we go along. Working through your emotional connection to things can help make those decisions; as you get stronger, it becomes less overwhelming.

Organizing Takes Grit

If you've ever refinished a piece of furniture, you know that there are different grit levels of sandpaper. Sandpaper with a low grit number is coarse and removes a lot of material, and a higher number grit is finer and continues to smooth what's left.

The same goes for organizing. You start with a rough sorting process which quickly helps you remove a lot of stuff you instantly know you don't want to keep. Each successive round refines the organizing process.

Level With Me

Each level starts with a question that asks you to make a decision. Decisions get more challenging at each level, but you can do it because you have been training. Each lower-level decision has built up your decision-making muscles so you can handle it.

Following the levels in order is best until organizing becomes second nature. Ready to go? Do you want to start in the kitchen or under the bathroom sink?

Key Takeaway

Organizing is a series of decisions; you must start small and build up to the tougher ones. Like working out, the more you do it, the stronger you become at deciding what to keep and let go.

Chapter 10

To Keep or Not to Keep? That is the Question

It's much easier for people to help declutter someone else's home because they don't have emotions invested in someone else's stuff. A friend will come over one morning to help, start picking up things, ask, "Keep?" and expect a quick answer so you can finish and go out to lunch. "That's the whole problem!" you think. "I can't decide." And suddenly, you're anxious, your motivation is gone, and you can't even decide where to go to lunch.

I guarantee you can make decisions about some things. You keep your birth certificate; you do not keep last week's grocery advertisements. You keep the new pot you just bought; you throw away the one with the broken handle, which is why you bought the new one. And if you can't decide quickly about something, you skip it and go on to the next one, just like any other multiple-choice quiz.

Level One: Should It Stay or Should It Go?

Level one is a quick and easy way of roughly sorting things. It is easiest to start in a room like a kitchen or a bathroom where you are less likely to have emotional attachments and have a surface space you can clear to sort things into piles. Remember, we only do one drawer, cabinet, shelf, or surface at a time so that it won't be overwhelming.

The Two-Second Rule

You are making three piles: Keep, Let Go, and Maybe. Sometimes things are an instant "yes" or an instant "no." Hold or touch an item and instantly decide whether to keep it. **If you have to think about it for more than two seconds, put it into the Maybe pile and move on.** If you have to examine it to see if it's damaged or need to try it to see if it works, put it in the Maybe pile.

Let's say we are organizing the kitchen cabinet where you store your pots. Any pot or pan you use all the time is an instant yes. An instant no would be a heavily scratched or encrusted pan in the back of the cabinet that you won't use now that you have a new one. "Maybe" would be things you have duplicates or multiples of that you must examine to determine which to keep.

Keep Calm and Move On

All you are doing is making instant decisions that are easy for you. If it's not easy and you can't decide, put it in the Maybe pile. You don't need to worry about keeping too much stuff or what you will do with it if you don't keep it. You don't want to get sidetracked by indecision. When you use the Two-Second Rule, you won't feel rushed to make an irrevocable decision.

Level Two: Sell, Donate, or Trash?

In Level Two, you only decide what to do with what you just decided to let go. For this level, you need two or three garbage bags (Trash, Recycle, and possibly Shred if you are sorting papers) and at least two boxes for Sell and Donate. I recommend boxes instead of plastic bins so you can use the plastic for what you are keeping.

Pick up each thing in the "Let It Go" pile from level one and decide Trash, Recycle, Shred, Donate, or Sell. Remember, you only look at the things you already decided not to keep. If you regret a decision and don't want to get rid of it, put it back into Level One's Maybe pile.

If you can't decide between selling or donating in two seconds, put it in the Sell box and move on. We are working out your decision-making muscles, and you are still a lightweight. The trick is to keep moving and not get caught up in emotion, indecision, or anything that will slow your momentum. Whatever doesn't sell, you'll donate later.

Level Three: Is This the Wrong Stuff?

In Level Three, the decisions get tough. You must look at your Maybe pile and decide whether something is the "wrong stuff." Use your "brain" (aka your phone) to get information, and if you don't know what something is, use Google Lens with your phone's camera to identify it.

- Check out the condition:
  - Is it worn or damaged?
  - Does it work?
  - Has it expired?
- Compare it to others:
  - Do I have another one?
  - Do I need more than one?
  - Does it have different features?
- Research price and availability:
  - Can I get it again if I need it? How soon, and for how much?
  - Is it worth saving and taking up space?
  - Can it be repaired for less money than buying it new?

- Examine its usefulness:
  - How and when do you use it?
  - Do I have a reasonable substitute?
  - Is there an app on my phone that can do the same thing?
- Determine relevance:
  - Does it fit?
  - Is it my style?
  - Am I still interested in it?
- Sort through papers:
  - Is it irrelevant or expired?
  - Do I have the information saved elsewhere?
  - Am I required to keep it?
- Protect your mental health:
  - Does it trigger a negative emotional reaction?
  - Is there a benefit besides documenting my history?
  - Can I keep a small part if I can't let it go completely?
  - Can someone else store it for me?

If you decide to Let Go, put it into the appropriate bag or box. After evaluating the whole Maybe pile, you might still have items you're not sure about. That's fine. There will be another round. On to level four!

Key Takeaway

Organize one shelf, drawer, or surface at a time to avoid being overwhelmed or frozen with emotion. If you can't make a decluttering decision in two seconds, pass over it and keep going. It will become clearer what to do with an item as you progress.

Chapter 11

The Heart of Organizing

Once you know what you're keeping, the decluttering decisions become storage decisions. At Level Four, you decide where things go and how to store them, which might impact what to do with items if you are still on the fence. This level is the heart of organizing; by the end, you have made all the tough decisions. Then, Level Five is the highly sorted, visually pleasing Pinterest-worthy level of organization that comes last after all the hard work is done. It's okay if you don't get to that level, and you can still feel very proud about what you've accomplished in Level Four.

Level Four: Where Does This Go?

By this time, you have made dozens of decisions, and it's been a while since you made those initial snap decisions of what to keep.

Since this is the stage where you figure out how much space you need for the things you want to store, take a quick "Level Three look" at the Keep pile to ensure you still want everything there. You might find it possible to reduce even more because all that decision-making has strengthened you mentally. Sometimes looking at what's in the Keep pile helps you decide about anything left in the Maybe pile.

Which of These Things Belong Together?

So, how do you decide where things go? First, think of Sesame Street. Which of these things belong together? Which of these things are kind of the same?

If there's something obviously out of place from the rest, put that in the laundry basket. For example, if you find an insulated travel mug hanging out with the water bottles while organizing the water bottle shelf, the travel mug goes in the laundry basket, even if you know where it's supposed to go. Leaving the task at hand may lead you to get distracted and not come back, so wait to put away the insulated mug until you finish with the water bottles.

Now, do you have all the water bottles? You want to collect them in one place, so you know how many you have and how much space you need to store them. Are there any on the counter, in the dishwasher, with the lunch boxes? Don't forget the kids' rooms and their backpacks! When you find more, quickly sort so you know exactly what you are keeping.

Do They All Fit?

Next, do the water bottles all fit on the shelf where they were, and if so, does it make sense to keep them there? If the answer is yes to both, you're golden! Just put them back. If you have extra space, look again at the bottles in the Maybe pile and see if you can keep some more and eliminate the rest. You may discover that keeping a neatly arranged shelf is worth more than extra water bottles.

If the water bottles don't all fit in the space where you took them out but still go in the kitchen, put them aside for a bit and continue to the next space in the kitchen where you suspect they will fit. After you've done more of the kitchen, it becomes clearer where there is space to rearrange things. Or you may want to downsize the bottle collection to fit the available space.

If you decide that the water bottles would be better stored in another room (the mudroom, for example), put them together in a bag and put them in the laundry basket so you can relocate them when you are done organizing where you are.

Form Follows Function, and Pretty Comes Later

The end of level four is arranging everything neatly in the drawer, shelf, cabinet, closet, or surface you've just spent time sorting. For now, use what you have for drawer organizers and containers. Form follows function, and pretty comes later. Most people already have things to use, so look around the house and be creative. All you are looking for is the right shape and size. After you know what you need, take the dimensions of the space you are working on and look for containers that maximize that space.

I do not recommend buying new containers before you know what they will be used for and where they will be located. The exception to this is plastic shoe boxes. You can keep shoe boxes on hand, but they are not all created equal. Shoe boxes are great for shoes and many things you store on shallow shelves in your cabinets and closets. You need to know the shelves' dimensions, so you can get shoe boxes that stack at least two high with their covers on and at least three across so you don't waste space on a shelf.

At the end of the book is a guide to buying containers and other products for organizing.

Nothing Is Permanent

Remember that nothing you arrange is permanent. You must live with it for a while to see if it works. Before you are done in a room, things may change containers and locations or whenever you organize another space.

I use a temporary labeling system of blue painter's tape and Sharpie; it's cheap, quick, and easily removed when necessary. You can go back and use a label maker later if you want. I rarely use label makers when working with my clients because I work by the hour, and I don't think they want to pay me for the extra minutes it takes to spell out, cut, peel, and affix the label. Blue tape and Sharpie get the job done if you don't have the time, energy, or money to use a label maker.

Level Five: How Far Do I Want to Go?

You've seen the images: Stylish, color-coordinated containers and labels designed to go with a modern, minimalist, sleek room. Beautiful desks impractically arranged with matching accessories and file folders organized by color for each category. Clothes organized by size, color, and season on matching hangers. Shoes stacked in identical plastic shoeboxes with pictures and descriptions displayed on the front.

Do you need all this to feel a space is neat and organized? No, but if you have the time, money, energy, and inclination to go that far, knock yourself out! If you don't, you are still a success!

Level Five can be done immediately or anytime later. It's the pretty, if not practical, organization you see in After pictures and on HGTV.

However, if something is a pain to remove, use, and put back, you will still have a mess, no matter how pretty the container is. If you can't keep up with the sorting and storing system, what's the point? The most important thing is that the containers and accessories help you maintain the level of organization you've accomplished.

Key Takeaway

Function comes first, and pretty comes later. As long as things are neatly arranged so you can find what you need and put them away easily, you can still feel organized and proud of your work, even if your home doesn't look like HGTV.

Chapter 12

Don't Just Stand There

An organizing session can last five minutes to five hours, so saying you don't have time is not an excuse. Rarely will you ever have more than five hours of uninterrupted time to organize; even if you do, five hours is usually the max your brain and body can take. You don't want to overdo it and not be able to move the next day.

Short Sessions

If you have physical limitations or ADHD and get distracted easily, you will have to do things in smaller chunks, which might mean you get less done in a day than you'd like. Don't let that stop you.

Start thinking about what you can do in shorter sessions and still feel progress. You can organize your coffee mug shelf while waiting for your coffee to brew or organize the silverware while heating your lunch in the microwave. You can organize your purse in the car while you are waiting in the carpool line or organize your car while your kid is in a piano lesson.

Prioritize

Many people need help with the executive function skills of initiating and prioritizing tasks. It's hard to get started or even know what to do first. As if you were setting your exercise schedule for the week, I suggest you schedule out when and what you'll be organizing this week ahead of time. Tell yourself, "I'm just going to organize this one drawer." That will get you started, and the momentum will keep you going, so you might be able to do more than you realize.

Aggravation is Motivation

Start by taking care of things that aggravate you when you prepare for the day. For example, if you have to dig through your drawer to get to the "good" underwear or take time to find a pair of matching socks, do a dresser drawer that day. If you can't find a sharp razor or get to a Q-Tip quickly, organize a cabinet or drawer in the bathroom. Couldn't find an umbrella or a coat that fit this morning? The coat closet is what you should work on next. I'm not saying to do it right then when you get aggravated. Just make a note (mental, physical, or digital) that this is the area you will work on later today.

The Right Time to Organize

Here are some ideas of what you can organize whether you have a few minutes or hours. You may want to write a list of your own, so you don't waste time deciding what to do when you have the opportunity.

- 5 minutes: shower, silverware, earrings, purse, glove box
- 10 minutes: bathroom drawer, sock drawer, first aid kit, board games, utensils
- 15 minutes: office supplies, art supplies, video game station, email, contacts
- 30 minutes: shoes, cookware, pet supplies, cleaning supplies, make-up,
- 1 hour: laundry room, desk, towels, bedding, sheets, bookcase, bar
- 2 hours: files, holiday decorations, pantry, bathroom, display cabinet
- 3 hours: bedroom closet, playroom, office, gift closet, party supplies
- 4 hours: backyard, storage unit, set up a room
- 5 hours: transform a room, half the garage, or basement

Prepare to Avoid Distractions

Your mind may swirl while you are organizing and distract you by remembering everything else you have to do, worrying about how to handle a situation, or ruminating on how you could have handled it better. Physical sensations like hunger, thirst, tiredness, or pain can make you less productive, so you should take care of yourself first before you organize. Ensure you are well rested, fed, hydrated, and caffeinated if necessary.

Arm for Battle

Just as if you were getting ready to go to work, go to the bathroom, take your medicine, fill a water bottle, and pack snacks. If your blood sugar goes too low, you won't be able to make decisions which means the end of organizing for the day. Don't forget to drink! While you're working, make time for "hydration and elimination." If you are physically uncomfortable, you will be less effective, and you don't want to hit a stumbling block by associating organizing with being uncomfortable.

Do What it Takes to Keep Working

When your mind won't stay focused, acknowledge the intrusion and then do what it takes for you to keep working:

- Write a to-do list
- Set the alarm
- Enter an appointment in your calendar
- Schedule a reminder
- Send a text
- Make a call
- Play music

Do whatever you need to quiet your mind without physically leaving the spot. You can do all that on your phone, which should always be charged and nearby.

In addition to supplying knowledge at your fingertips, your phone provides powerful tools to help with executive function and organization:

- Notes
- Calendar
- Clock
- Message
- Mail
- Phone
- Maps
- Camera / Google Lens

Lights, Camera, Organize!

The camera is helpful because you can take pictures of things you must do instead of writing them out. In school, a frequent IEP accommodation is taking a picture of the board instead of writing assignments in a planner. At my house, we keep a list on the whiteboard in the kitchen of what we need and then take a picture of the list before we go grocery shopping. Plus, you use the camera to access Google Lens, which helps you identify an object to decide where it goes.

Go Old School

If you don't know how to use these apps yet or don't want to be even more distracted by having your phone with you, bring a pen and notebook to get thoughts out of your head and onto paper, where you will deal with them later.

Reward Yourself for Results

When you complete an organizing job, reward yourself with a treat or whatever motivates you to continue organizing. I like to post on Facebook and get a dopamine high when I see all the "likes." But only reward yourself when you complete the job because it's not done until you follow through.

Key Takeaway

You don't have to wait for a big block of time to organize; you can organize something no matter how much time you have. Prepare for distractions and reward yourself for motivation.

Chapter 13

Follow Through

All your excellent work editing and organizing will go to waste if you leave what's left over sitting on the floor, back of the cabinet, or bottom of the closet. Keep an eye on the time, and don't start working on another shelf, drawer, or cabinet if you don't have enough time to take care of what you've done already.

Whether you have five minutes or five hours to organize that day, use the last fifth of the time to follow through. That means if you have five minutes to organize the silverware drawer, leave the last minute to follow through with whatever you took out that's not going back. That's enough time to get things to the trash, recycle bin, donation box, or magic laundry basket (more on that later.)

If you know where something goes and have time, you can throw it in the right drawer even if you can't put it away nicely. At least it's in the right place, and now you know which drawer to organize tomorrow while you're waiting for the microwave. Done is better than perfect.

Trash

If something is too big to fit in the trash, take it to the curb and call for a bulky item pickup. If you can't carry junk to the curb or need it gone sooner, call 1-800-GOT-JUNK or a hauling company. They will pick up your junk wherever it is on your property and charge you for the space it takes up in their truck. If you can't make the call now, schedule the phone call in your calendar, so you don't forget. Nothing is more satisfying than getting rid of junk, even if you have to pay.

Recycling

Metal is easily recycled. If it doesn't fit in the recycling bin, you can leave it at the curb, and, as if by magic, a metal collector in a truck will come by and take it away. You don't even have to call someone.

Think realistically about whether you will haul bags to the recycling center to redeem glass jars, bottles, and cans. There are fewer recycling centers than there used to be, so it may not be worth your time. You can save the earth and save yourself a trip by offering them to someone who needs the money more than you do. I post on a free site, and someone with an enterprising kid usually picks them up from me.

Cardboard and paper are easily recycled in the bin. If you have boxes suitable for moving or shipping, you may want to offer them on a free site before filling your bin.

Shredding

If you don't own or can't borrow a shredder, places like the UPS Store and Staples will shred your stuff for you for a price. Office Depot will pick up your shredding at an even higher price. Just be aware that the bags may sit for a week or more before the contents go to a third-party shredder. Sometimes there are free community "shred events" when you can take your papers to a shredding truck and watch them as they are shredded. Look at shredit.com or shrednations.com. To reduce the need for shredding, consider going green and having statements sent to you online only, and rip up junk mail as soon as you bring it in from the mailbox.

Donating

Get into the habit of bagging or boxing donations right away. Take them to your car or front door so you are not tempted to reconsider your decision. Then go to the donation center or schedule a pickup.

I have a client who reuses old suitcases to take donations for drop-off. She packs the stuff in there so she doesn't have to see them and empties them when she arrives. Don't forget you have boxes or suitcases full of donations in the car. I have been guilty of letting donations rattle around for weeks in the back of my car.

At the end of the book, there are resources for finding a charity in your area that accepts donations and supports a cause important to you. It will make your life easier if you always call first to find out if the charity does pick-ups and precisely what they take and don't take. If you wouldn't buy it, they won't take it. There are certain things that they don't take anymore, especially since the pandemic when charities were inundated.

Many charities schedule their pick-ups online. If you are in a hurry, don't wait to schedule the appointment until you finish sorting, and you will be motivated to finish sooner with a pickup deadline in mind.

Hidden Money

I always tell my clients that they will find money when they organize, whether it's a few coins, an envelope full of cash, or even a bond that has been misplaced for years. You never know where someone has stashed money, so before you donate anything, remember to look through all the pockets, under the mattress, underneath drawers, and inside boxes to find any hidden money.

The $100 Sunburn

If you're thinking about having a garage sale, don't bother. Most people I know make about $100 and still need to take most of their stuff to the donation center. Plus, they end up with a bad sunburn. Better to donate them and get a tax deduction. Or list them for free (unless it's a dining room buffet or entertainment center. You can't even give them away.)

Love It or List It

Take pictures and list things to give away on Facebook Marketplace and free groups like Buy Nothing, Offer Up, or Craig's List -- wherever you are comfortable. Keep in mind some sites like eBay, Poshmark, and Depop charge a commission. To sell quality children's clothes or furniture, investigate consignment shops. At the end of the book, I have included resources for selling unwanted items.

Key Takeaway

Every time you organize, leave time to follow through with the things you remove: Put away, take to the car or front door, list online, take to the trash. Otherwise, they will become another pile of clutter.

PART 3

Maintaining Balance

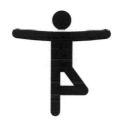

Chapter 14

Done Is Better Than Perfect

I am a perfectionist. I am critical of everything I experience that I know can be better, whether it's a room arrangement, a piece of writing, a show, an event, or how a company is run. It's okay if it's your job to point out things that can be improved, and it may be motivating if you're trying to achieve excellence at your job or in competition. But if you are critical of yourself to the point where you feel the need to be perfect or otherwise feel like a failure, that is perfectionism, and it's not a good thing.

Perfectionism

Perfectionism is related to anxiety and OCD. If you procrastinate regularly, you may be experiencing perfectionism. You might resist starting a task because you're afraid you'll be unable to complete it perfectly.

As a student, I would put off writing school papers or working on big projects, waiting for a big enough chunk of time to exclusively focus on it so I could do it to the best of my ability. Of course, that time didn't materialize until the night before the assignment was due, along with an overdose of anxiety steadily building since the assignment was announced. Some of my best work happened under pressure between midnight and an 8:00 am class, but I would always think how much better it would have been if I had had more time.

Recovering Perfectionist

A better term for me now is "recovering perfectionist." As a mom, I have learned over the years that life comes at you so fast that there's no way to have the luxury of doing everything exactly how you want it in the time you have to do it. You can't wait for a big chunk of time to start a project so you can do it right. There will always be demands on your time and attention. Setbacks, curveballs, detours, and distractions are just what life is. My mantra now is "done is better than perfect."

Organizing Is Not a "One and Done"

No one - repeat after me - no one finds it easy to organize. Organizing is an ongoing process that gets easier as you use the tools and tips you learn as you go. Some days it's easier than others. Life happens, moods change, and energy wanes. As I write this, my house is in flux as we reorganized my kid's bedroom to accommodate a new cat.

But organizing is an active process, not a static state. The following week my house was back to normal, even better because I could donate things that cluttered my kid's room and more when I reorganized the garage to accommodate what was left. That's how it goes. Nobody expects you to have everything completely organized at once and maintain that forever. As things in your life change, so will your organization.

Organized, Not Staged

It is unrealistic to expect that your home, if you are actively living there, will always look like HGTV, with everything put away and guest-ready. If that's your idea of an organized home, you will constantly be disappointed in yourself.

That's not what organized looks like; it's what "staged" looks like.

Nobody lives in a staged home. It may look nice, but people are not always comfortable in a home where guests are afraid to put anything down. However, you can expect your house to look staged at a particular time (like the start of a party).

You will reach a point where your home can look like that within an hour or two because you have created the space and the system to do it. Everything will have a place where it can be put away quickly, and I don't mean shoved in a closet or stuffed in the oven!

Remember, as long as you've removed the wrong stuff and created space for everything else, you're still organized, even if your rooms are messy at any given moment.

You just haven't invited anyone over yet.

Leftovers

After you've organized a space and everything is neatly arranged, some stuff still belongs somewhere else. What do you do if you don't have time to put it away where it goes, or if you don't know where it goes, or even know what it is? That's why things often stay on the floor, on a table, or hide where they don't belong.

The Junk Drawer

Some people have a junk drawer for little things, but I think that's a waste of prime real estate. Drawers, like shelf space, are gold in the organizing business. I keep a junk shoebox in my laundry room for little things I feel I should keep but have no idea what they go with, where I should put them, or the time and energy to run right out and get them there. Examples are:

- a piece of plastic that belongs to something, but I can't figure out what.

- a spare part that I haven't made a home for yet.
- a screw that belongs in the garage, but it's raining, and I don't want to go outside.

Like my orphan socks shoebox, I know to look there first if I'm looking for something little which isn't where it's supposed to be.

But what do you do if it doesn't fit in a shoebox?

The Magic Laundry Basket

The magic laundry basket is where you will put things in your Keep pile that don't belong in the space you are organizing and are too big to fit in a junk shoebox.

Laundry baskets work because they are readily available, easily identified by shape or color, and have handles, so they're easy to carry.

Bins, tubs, and boxes may all look the same, and the label (if it has one) may not be easy to read. But if you say, "the white laundry basket," everyone knows exactly what you mean and can identify it from across the room. This laundry basket should only be used for organizing, even if it sometimes sits empty. It should be a different color or shape than the one you use for laundry so you can easily distinguish it.

Making the Rounds

The laundry basket is a bonanza when you have to tidy up quickly because company is coming (or you have to clean for the housekeeper!) Take the laundry basket with you whenever you are organizing or cleaning up. If you find something that doesn't belong in the room where you are, put it in the laundry basket.

Don't Leave!

I know you're dying to put that random spoon back in the kitchen, but I don't want you to get distracted by leaving. You may never come back! It can stay in the laundry basket until you are done in the room and go to the next room you need to tidy.

Take it With You

If you're ready for the next room, take the basket with you and start, or leave it there for the next session. Making the rounds and tidying up with the laundry basket is a good use of a 15-30 minute organizing session.

When you get to the next room, look for things in the basket that belong in that room and put them away. Again, whatever doesn't belong in that room goes into the basket.

If you don't have time to put things away where they go (or don't know where that is), they stay in the laundry basket until you get them to the right place. Then, if someone is looking for something, they will know to look in the laundry basket first.

The same stuff mustn't live in the basket for over a week. If you still don't know where it goes after you've made the rounds, I would put it in a miscellaneous box in the garage or basement (if you have one) and schedule a time to revisit it when you have time for an extended session. Done is better than perfect!

Key Takeaway

Organizing is an ongoing process that gets easier with practice, and practice makes progress, not perfect. If you wait to do something until you can do it perfectly, you'll never get anything done.

Chapter 15

Crap Equilibrium

Years ago, my best friend Jenn and I decided to have a two-family garage sale. Since her house had more foot traffic, it was in her driveway, and my husband and I brought over our stuff for what has now become known as "the crap exchange." Jen coined that lovely phrase because instead of selling our crap to other people, the result was exchanging a lot of it with each other. One person's trash is another person's treasure, so stuff in her garage ended up in my house and vice versa. That's when I came up with the idea of "Crap Equilibrium."

When you get something new, whether bought, gifted, thrifted, or handed down, you must give up something for every item you bring home so your home can remain in balance.

There must be an equilibrium because you only have so much space. You cannot keep adding without giving something up, or you'll end up with drawers that won't close and an avalanche falling on you every time you open a door. Instead of bringing you joy, your things will only bring you aggravation. When you practice crap equilibrium and regularly edit what you own, you will lose pounds of excess stuff weighing you down and regain valuable real estate (storage space) for new acquisitions. You can still bring home treasures without your home looking like trash.

Just One Space at a Time

Making room for your finds requires you to organize what you already have. I know you think the phrase "organize what you have" is overwhelming. I'm not suggesting a big project to go through your entire home. I'm encouraging you to make space by going through just one shelf, cabinet, drawer, closet, wall, or room at a time — wherever something new is going — and getting rid of just one thing to make room for the new thing. If you can get rid of more, that's even better.

Keep Your Best, Reduce the Rest

Right away, go through the cabinet, drawer, closet, or room where the new thing belongs, scan it, and see if there is at least one thing in that space to let go. Look for ripped, stained, frayed, worn out, damaged, outdated, obsolete, or outgrown things. Those are the easiest decisions to make. Then look at the quality of what's left. You deserve nice things. Keep your best and reduce the rest.

Use it or Lose It

Clothes in the laundry, dishes in the sink and dishwasher, and everything left out on the counters, couches, tables, and floors are most likely used all the time. What is left in the cabinets, drawers, and closets is used less. If you still need help deciding what to give up, the things at the bottom or back of the drawers, cabinets, or closets are an excellent place to start. Look for duplicates and multiples of things. If you only like big coffee mugs and reach for those each morning, you don't need little ones cluttering your shelf. People will always choose their favorite thing over another. So even if those Ticonderoga No. 2 pencils and blue-capped Bic pens are perfectly usable, they will forever take up valuable space if your family prefers the mechanical pencils and click pens.

You Replaced It for a Reason

Don't leave things you just replaced sitting at the back of the shelf, the bottom of the drawer, or stuffed in the closet. The lack of space there will make it difficult to get to the things you use and impossible to put them back away. It will make your life more difficult, which is ironic because the new things you get are supposed to bring you joy. Even if they do fit, why keep them? You are always going to use the new one you brought home instead. Get into the habit of bagging or boxing things up to give away and take care of them immediately so you are not tempted to reconsider your decision.

Close Only Counts in Horseshoes and Organizing

If you bring home something out of season (from an after-holiday sale, for example) or for occasional use (like camping gear), you may know where it goes, but it's not easily accessible without having to do ten things first. If you can't open a container quickly because it's too high up or there are other things stacked on top, you have no choice but to store your new item as close as possible to the container so you see it and won't forget about it when it's time to go through the collection. When you see everything together, it is easier to pick out your favorites and let go of the ones you don't care as much about.

Hit or Miss

When you bring home clothes, toys, games, or books for someone in your family, wait until they can actively receive them, like a gift. If you dump it in their room, it will likely sit around for a while until *you* do something with it since people will usually only take ownership if they have seen it, tried it on, or tried it out and let you know they like it. If you don't hand it to them and watch, you won't know if it's a hit or a miss. If it's a hit, have them put it away. If they like something but don't care enough to put it away, then there's no use in keeping it because you think they might like it someday.

The Gift Closet

A dedicated gift closet is a convenient way to save money and give gifts throughout the year without going to the store or shopping online for a present at the moment you need it. All year, you shop for bargains, go to garage sales and thrift stores, and pick up things for free. Don't care for a gift, lost the receipt, or it's too late to return it? Put it in the gift closet. Then when there is an occasion to bring a present, you go shopping in your closet and don't forget about the gifts you buy throughout the year. The gift closet also stores gift bags, wrapping paper, tissue, shred, ribbons, tape, scissors, cards, and everything else you need for gift-giving. Everything is in one place, so you don't have to search for wrapping supplies.

Don't be like my mom, who, while we were opening Christmas presents, would run back to her room with the wrapping paper from the presents we just opened to "wrap" more presents (without tape) because she couldn't find her supplies to wrap them ahead of time.

Keep Your Side of the Street Clean

I hear from clients that it is impossible to declutter because a spouse keeps bringing things home, or their spouse has a room so filled with stuff that they can't stand to look at it, so they keep the door shut. Yet there are rooms in the rest of the home that need organizing that have nothing to do with the spouse's unwillingness to give things up.

I advocate for people to have a space where no one nags them to declutter. There's a saying, "Keep your side of the street clean." What's on the other side of the street is their responsibility, so focus on yours. And who knows? Once your spouse sees the results of your organizing, they may be motivated to declutter and organize their space too.

Key Takeaway

Continuing to organize one space at a time will keep your home in balance. Every time you bring something home, look through what you already have and let at least one thing go.

Chapter 16

In With the New

It's incredible how much stuff we acquire. Retail therapy is a way of life for some people. For me, going to flea markets and thrifting (as my daughter calls shopping in second-hand stores) has been a family tradition since I was a kid. Over the years, I've brought home so many finds from the thrift store and things I picked up for free that I can't tell you where they came from.

The only downside to bringing things home is having to organize and make space so you can put them away. Here are some tips I've learned that can help you integrate what you bring home into what you already have.

Books

When you bring home a book, give yourself a few months. If you haven't picked it up by then --and by picked up, I mean read and not just moved somewhere -- pass it on, or pass on a book you already read, so you can keep crap equilibrium and not overwhelm your bookshelf or nightstand.

Clothes

If you didn't before, try on every piece of clothing you bring home the same day. If it doesn't fit now, pass it on unless it's fur, leather, silk, or some valuable fabric. If you are keeping a garment, you might want to wash it first, then hang it up, fold it, and put it away. While the drawers or closet doors open, quickly scan to see if you have anything similar you would pass over for the new garment. For example, if you have a few black jackets, see if you like the new one better. Whichever one you like better is the one you'll pull out when it's time to wear a black jacket.

I understand keeping jackets in different styles and sizes. If you now have two black blazers of the same size, only so many hangers fit in your closet, so may the best jacket win!

Hangers

If you are a fashionista with closet space to support your habit, I recommend buying an extra package or two of thin felt hangers. I strongly suggest you do not pick up those fat plastic hangers or wire dry-cleaning hangers I see people giving away. It is lousy to be aggravated first thing in the morning by hangers that don't slide and clothes that slide off hangers. For heavy coats and suits, I like to use wood hangers. For everything else, I like felt hangers. Having them all the same color is nice, but it's up to you. Hangers seem to be a hot commodity in my house, so I bought different colors and styles for each family member. That way, if I run out of hangers in my room, I can see by their closet who poached mine.

Hand Me Downs

When you get a bag of hand-me-downs for your kids, dump it all, go through it immediately, and put the things you don't want back into the bag for donation. Then go through the rest, sort by size, and only have the kids look immediately at what they could wear. Kids are just as overwhelmed as adults when having to make decisions on what to keep. If they are not excited about it and don't need it, put it back in the donation bag. If it doesn't fit now, put it in a container, and when they reach the right size, go through those clothes at that time.

Collectibles

There is no use keeping a collection if you don't have a place to show it off or space and a method to store what's not on display safely.

Otherwise, it is clutter that will probably get ruined if someone else (who doesn't care about it as much as you) packs it up.

If you have a collection of value (like stamps, coins, baseball cards, records, movie memorabilia, etc.), find a resource to appraise each piece and a solid plan on selling it when it's time. At the end of the book, I have listed a few resources for appraising and selling specific collections.

So, when you want to pick up that angel figurine to add to your collection, make sure that there will be room for it on the shelf and that you like it as much as or better than whatever you have now. A collection can become overwhelming clutter unless you occasionally go through it and exchange a new find for one you could live without. You might even discover that you liked the new one because you already have the same one! In that case, keep the one in the best shape and discard the duplicate.

Yona's Elephants

My mother-in-law had many elephant figurines, and they were everywhere in her house, and people would give her elephants as gifts to add to her collection. Many years into my marriage, she told me that she really didn't like elephants and liked horses instead. The only reason she had so many elephants is that someone gave her an elephant once, and someone else saw it, assumed she liked elephants and brought her another one.

Over the years, friends would see elephants and think of Yona, so she received them as gifts for every occasion. She thought, like many others, you can't get rid of a gift, so the collection kept growing.

When she passed, I kept a few cool ones and distributed the rest of her collection to friends and relatives who wanted one. I found three of the same silver-colored elephant stamped with GOP, which was amusing since she was an extremely dedicated Democrat and probably never noticed the symbol. I gave those GOP elephants to Republican friends.

Furniture

If you pick up a piece of furniture, know that it will probably take some work to incorporate it into your home, and if you don't have the time or the energy – don't get it! If it is replacing something, make sure that it fits in your car and your room BEFORE you pick it up, and ideally, take the thing it is replacing out first before bringing the new thing home. If it falls into the black hole of "Later" (meaning, your garage or basement), chances are by the time you look at it again, you might realize it's not going to work in the space you intended, and it took up valuable real estate all that time for no reason.

If the furniture is a "project," make sure you know what you are getting yourself into. If spending your free time covered in sawdust and paint and smelling like turpentine is not something you know you enjoy, or if it's the middle of summer and it's too hot out, and you won't get to it until winter when it's too cold/windy/dark, then don't get it – unless you're very good at refinishing furniture and this hobby has become a money-making business – in which case, I've got an antique table rotting outside, which you are welcome to take away.

Holiday Decorations

Store the decorations you accumulate throughout the year as close as possible to the ones you already have so you remember you have them when the holiday rolls around.

After you pull everything out and decorate, look at what you're not using. Is it damaged? Throw it away. Would you use it another year for a different theme or location? Keep it. Are you not using it this year because you like the new stuff better? That's what you can get rid of for crap equilibrium. I'm not talking about the sentimental things your kids made in school. You can keep those things even if they are falling apart; you don't have to put them out, but it's nice to see those memories every year. If you don't have room for everything, take photos and keep just your favorites.

Kitchenware

If you're like me, you go into a store for one thing you need and end up with a shopping cart full of things for the kitchen you like better than what you already have. But your kitchen cabinets and drawers can only hold so much until you are aggravated whenever you try to open them. To keep equilibrium, you are going to have to edit.

When you make your morning coffee, you probably use the new oversized mug from Starbucks instead of the little chipped one you've had forever, right? It's probably out instead of in the cabinet because it's your favorite. Whatever sits in the back of the cabinets and the bottom of the drawers are "back-ups" and the first to go when you get something new. Then the new things become your favorites, and the stuff you now use all the time becomes backup.

Gadgets

As for gadgets, when was the last time you made a melon ball? Pitted a cherry? Have you made veggies into spaghetti? Stuck a spout into an orange and drank the juice? How many people in your house cut grapefruits at the same time? Which peeler is the one that doesn't give you blisters? Life is too short to be aggravated by dull peelers and ridiculous gadgets cluttering your drawers. If you must use Google Lens to identify something, think of paring down your kitchen gadgets as saving your sanity. Then you can justify buying better stuff at the next Pampered Chef party you have to attend.

Framed Art and Signs

If a framed piece of art is new or will replace something you already have, make sure your partner, kid, or roommate likes it, then measure it to see if it fits in your wall space. Then get the tools you need and hang the art right away. If it sits, it is likely to break before you can put it up, and then you've been decorating your baseboard for no reason, and you will have shards of glass decorating your floor until they find your bare foot.

Make sure you have the wall space if it's a sign for a specific space like the kitchen or laundry room. If it's for a holiday, and the holiday rolls around, and it doesn't get put up, pass it on while it's still that holiday season.

Tableware

You may have many tablecloths, napkins, and napkin rings, but you probably only use the same ones over and over. When you bring home a tablecloth or napkins, check out the condition of the ones you already have. If you don't like the color or quality or don't own a table that size, put it straight into the giveaway bag. If you are like me and can't be bothered working on stains, toss it with anything ripped or frayed. If you want to save one for a picnic, when did you last go on one? You can put it in the picnic basket, so it doesn't add to the clutter in the tablecloth drawer.

If you still have multiple similar tablecloths, think of any occasion where you would use all of them at once. Is there a reason you would pick one over another (Higher quality? Prettier fabric? Family heirloom?) That might help narrow it down. You will probably find that you can let some go or need another size, shape, or color.

As for napkin rings, put the new set alongside the others to see which ones you like best. Then tie each set together with a ribbon instead of leaving them loose in the drawer because if you can't find all of them, you won't use them, and then what's the point in cluttering your drawer?

Suppose you have a single napkin or napkin ring without a match. You can repurpose it, or attach a note if it holds significant sentimental value, like it was always on the Thanksgiving table growing up. Even though I do not use them, in my drawer, I have a napkin embroidered by my grandmother and a monogrammed napkin ring belonging to my great-grandmother, which reminds me of them every time I set the table.

Carol's Christmas Napkin Ring

I have a single Christmas napkin ring from my mother, which holds a memory. When I was a young adult, my mom found a napkin ring on the floor, carelessly put it over a candlestick, and forgot about it. Later that night, she lit a candle, and as it burned, the napkin ring caught fire, which burned a hole in the table, and the house was filled with smoke. The walls had to be repainted, even the mural in my bedroom that my friend painted for my 13th birthday. This little napkin ring reminds me of that mural whenever I open the drawer. But if I hadn't written this down, no one would know why I had it, and it would probably be thrown away along with that piece of family history.

So, if you have only one piece left of a set, but you're keeping it because it's very sentimental, label it to let whoever goes through your things know there isn't a match, and write a note about why you kept it.

Towels

Towels take up a lot of room, especially if old ones get pushed to the back every time you get a new one. Wouldn't it be nice to have your towel shelf look like it belongs in a store and not go through the pile to find the one you like? Towels are easy to declutter. If it's threadbare, faded, bleach-stained, frayed, an ugly color, or too small to dry an adult, cut them up for rags or give them to an animal shelter. Unless you need one of them to dye your hair, you deserve big, fluffy, soft towels, and you don't have to keep the dreck. (That's Yiddish for rubbish or trash.)

Sheets

There is a debate on how many sets of sheets you need. You certainly don't need sheets for a bed size you don't have anymore. I would say that you need two sets for each bed in your home, one set for each air mattress or fold-out couch, and two sets of older twin-size sheets for each kid you send to camp (character sheets are perfect for this; my kids used the Charlie Brown sheets I had as a child.) If you don't use a top sheet, you can use the flat sheets from the sets for air mattresses and couches. All those fitted sheets where the elastic is shot? Gone. Ripped, stained, frayed? A no-brainer. Mismatched or a dated pattern? History. Yes, I know they're still useful, so rip one up for rags if you must, or keep some stored wherever you make forts. If you have a bunch of sheets left and not enough space to keep them all, put them to your cheek. The feel of them will tell you which ones you like best. Material, weave, and thread count make a difference, and most people have a preference. If you have more than enough, you don't need to keep anything that isn't your preference.

Pillows and Pillowcases

Keep four pillows for guests, or two if you can steal the rest from other beds. Each of our beds has two or three pillows per person, so we have extras for guests. Then go through your pillowcases and make sure they match the size pillows you have and go with the color scheme of your bedding. Get rid of anything that is ripped, stained, or frayed. If you have a choice, don't keep colors or patterns that don't match anything you have unless you need them for camp or trick-or-treating.

Blankets

Aside from what's already on your beds, you will need a sleeping bag, comforter, or blanket for each air mattress or pull-out couch. I like a cozy blanket for the couch and soft throws for each family member (including your dogs). If you have more than that and don't have the space, look for rips or stains to make your decision easier, and do the touch test on your cheek—no need to keep anything rough when such soft blankets are available. If you have a wool blanket, fold it and enclose it in a zipper bag to protect it from moths. If you have an electric blanket, it's best to store it folded in a zippered bag, so the cord and controls are contained and not spread out all over the shelf.

Office and School Supplies

I have had clients with enough school and office supplies to open a school or Staples store! Just because you can have it doesn't mean you should have it. You have limited drawer and shelf space, so make it count!

Do you need sheets of random-size labels and photo paper that come with a new printer? Most people don't, nor do they need 3-ring binders bigger than 2" unless they file brokerage statements. Is your tape dispenser sitting empty? If you are not committed to changing the roll as needed, disposable plastic dispensers take up less space.

If you go through your supplies often enough, you'll know what you need and won't spend too much when the back-to-school sales frenzy starts. I suggest going through your supplies during the first week in August, then again during Winter and Spring Break.

Let's start with the basics. Everyone has their favorite kind of pens and pencils.

If they like mechanical pencils, ensure you have the size they want and the lead that fits. If they like No. 2 Ticonderoga pencils, throw out the ones that are bitten, eraser-less, or shorter than your finger. If you keep them, no one will use them anyway.

Anything you keep around just because it's still usable, but is not as good as something else, will just take up precious space. If it's there, people will always choose their favorite. And if they have their favorite pen or pencil, they will enjoy school or work more.

Test your pens, markers, Hi-Liters, and Sharpies to see if they still have ink. You don't need broken crayons that not even a preschooler would use. No, you cannot melt them and make candles. It doesn't work, and when was the last time you made candles anyway? Sharpen colored pencils and see if the electric pencil sharpener even works. I find that little pencil sharpeners work better and take up less room.

Not all staplers are created equal, so try them out and pick the one(s) easiest to load that jams the least. Make sure mini staplers take regular-size staples. I bet you'll never bother buying mini-staple refills, so you may as well admit it and move on. I'm all about convenience and the least amount of aggravation.

Each kid should keep their supplies in a pencil case (They fit more than pouches and are easy to find in a backpack). In addition, you should have two more sets of supplies at home – one in a shared room for everyone to use and a secret stash for you so you don't have to search for a sharp pair of scissors or a stapler with staples.

You don't have to buy new packs of everything each year if you refine what you have throughout the year. However, getting a new box of crayons each August is still a treat. The Crayola 64-pack with the sharpener was my favorite birthday present growing up!

Key Takeaway

Make room to put away something new by organizing the space where it's going. If there's not enough space for everything, keep the favorite and let go of the least favorite because it won't get used anyway if you have a choice.

Chapter 17

Go to Your Room!

It's hard enough keeping your things organized. Keeping your kids' rooms organized can seem like you're being punished like Sisyphus, rolling the boulder up the hill only to have it roll back down and doing it again for eternity. For your mental health, teach your kids how to stay organized so they can find what they need and play, work, and sleep in a peaceful environment.

Set Them Up for Success

You don't want to be annoyed at your kids every time you walk into their room. Constantly telling them to "clean your room" will drive you crazy and won't get results unless you've set up the room in a way that makes it manageable.

Identify zones for certain activities: sleeping, dressing, doing homework, reading, playing, creating art, listening to music, etc., and create storage in each area, so everything has a home within reach and it's easy to keep neat.

You don't need a big room to create zones; in a small room, a zone can look like the closet, floor, bed, or door. Knowing what goes in each zone makes it easier to put things away because you can tell what does not belong there.

Sleeping Zone

The sleeping zone usually includes a bed, a nightstand, and a wastepaper basket. There should be as little as possible on the nightstand so things don't get knocked off when reaching for something, and it should have at least one drawer with a drawer organizer to keep things neat. If you go to bed with water, using a water bottle or insulated mug is best to avoid spills. The nightstand should be located near an outlet, so you can plug in a lamp, a phone, and an alarm clock or appliance (if necessary.) If you have a bunk bed, the bottom bunk might have a nightstand, and the top bunk might use a bedside shelf or nightstand tray.

If you want the bed made every morning, make sure it's easy to do with bedding that can be pulled up and smoothed out on every side. The ease of making the bed may be why kids choose not to have a top sheet, so you may want a duvet cover you can take off and wash if that's the case. It's hard to make a bed if it's against a wall, and the top bed of a bunk bed is even more challenging, so if that's what you have, understand the limitations and adjust your expectations accordingly. The only advantage is that pillows and stuffed animals may stay on the bed longer.

A little boy I used to watch could not sleep until all his stuffed animals were arranged on his bed. In the morning, they were all on the floor, behind the headboard, and under the bed, making it difficult and time-consuming to keep the bed neat.

When I had kids, I swore I would keep the stuffed animals and pillows in their rooms to a minimum, but my teenager still collects them! I just heard about bean bag covers for stuffed animals. Kids put all their stuffed animals inside, zip it up, and voila! It's a comfy, calming place to sit, read, or lie down. It's easy to unzip and get a different animal when they want to. They come in all sorts of shapes and sizes on Amazon.

Dressing Zone

The dressing zone usually includes a mirror, dresser, closet, hamper, and clothes storage. Check that drawers are aligned correctly and have a mechanism so they cannot be pulled all the way out. Kids will stop putting clothes away in a drawer if the drawer falls out when they open it or won't go back in when they try to close it. Sometimes you can skip the dresser if you have drawers or shelf space in the closet.

The best closet setup for a kid's room (really any room) has a high bar for long-hanging clothes and double bars, so little kids can hang their clothes on a bar they can reach. If you want kids to hang up clothes, use smaller hangers, so it's easier.

Ideally, the closet has low shelves, so you can store clothes folded as they are displayed in a store, and drawers or baskets for things like underwear and socks. If the closet doesn't have built-in shelves or drawers, you might want to get one of those hanging fabric closet organizers with small shelves/cubbies, which are easy for kids to use to put clothes away.

Shoes

You can use a hanging organizer for shoes if you have more hanging space or a shoe rack if you have more floor space than hanging space. You may want to keep shoes by the front door (or the door closest to the car) instead so you can put shoes on just before you leave the house.

The Hamper

It's best to have the hamper inside the closet or close to where your kid gets undressed. If you only have a hamper in the bathroom, you run the risk of kids leaving dirty clothes all over their room instead of taking them to the hamper in the bathroom. A hamper should be big enough so it won't overflow before laundry day and have handles so it can be easily carried to the laundry room, preferably by your kid if they are old enough. If they start throwing clean clothes in their hamper because they are too lazy to hang them up and put them away, then it's time they do their laundry instead of just bringing the hamper to the laundry room.

Clothes They Don't Wear Often

Seasonal clothes, special occasion clothes, and those of a different size can be stored in labeled plastic containers on a higher shelf. If your kid goes to summer camp, you can keep clothes, sheets, towels, and other things they exclusively take to camp every year in a plastic container on a closet shelf, so it is all together when you pack for camp.

You can also store "memory clothes" in a container on a shelf in the closet. Memory clothes are things they love or have a special meaning but don't wear anymore: T-shirts, uniforms, baby clothes, handmade costumes they outgrew, etc. If you are saving clothes for another generation, understand that even if they are washed, unseen stains can become visible with age and elastic crumbles. Maybe save one or two outfits from the age and pass on the rest so they can be worn and loved before they fall apart.

Homework / Creativity Zone

I have yet to meet a kid younger than high school who does homework at a desk in their room. Even though they don't use it for homework, a desk or a table with storage drawers can be used for drawing, writing, creating art, and playing games. It should be near a power outlet, especially if you allow a laptop or computer in their room.

Drawers are the key! If they aren't built into whatever you use as a desk, a plastic cart with drawers is necessary to hold school and art supplies. If you don't have drawer space, you can create storage by putting containers on shelves above or beside the desk or table.

Pulling out a drawer or putting something in an open container is easier than removing a top, taking something down, or opening a cabinet. And the easier it is to put something away, the more likely a kid will do it.

Reading Zone

If you want to foster a love for reading or writing, read to your kids, and if you have room, create the space in their room for you to read together and for them to read independently. At the very least, it should have a bookshelf they can reach, not too packed, so they can easily pull books out and put them away. Add a cozy chair or loveseat, a rug, and a reading lamp if there is space. If you make the space inviting, they will use it - If not for reading, then perhaps for listening to music, writing, coloring, etc.

Play Zone / Playroom

Wherever your kids play, whether in their room, the playroom, or the family room, stuff has to be stored at their height and easy to get out and put away. Shelves, cubbies, fabric boxes, plastic containers, baskets, drawers, cabinets, ottomans, and trunks are great as long as they are accessible, labeled with words or pictures, and easy to open and close. If a kid (or anyone really) has to work at putting something away, they won't. Or they won't do it quickly the first time you ask.

Keeping a playroom organized is an ongoing challenge. The toys the kids leave out are what they currently like playing with. If you don't have room to rotate toys so everything gets used, start editing with what they have outgrown or in which they no longer have an interest.

A good time to go through toys, games, and books is when you know there will be an influx of gifts, like holidays or birthdays. Visually teach kids that if their hand is closed holding on to something, they must first open it and let go to receive something new.

It would be best to go through the playroom with your kid(s), or they will carry a grudge forever. I've heard stories of giving away a toy, and later the kid sees it in the thrift store, so the parents panic and repurchase it.

Or it's hundreds of dollars for a mom to buy her favorite book set for her kids because her mom got rid of it without permission when she was a kid.

If you edit without your kid's input, maybe take the toys to Grandma's house so they can play with them there or put them in a box in the garage to go through later with them.

It's just as hard for them to give something away as it is for you. If you have toys they have outgrown, try using the name of a younger kid they adore (even if it goes to Goodwill instead). "You're getting so big and are playing with Barbies already. Should we give this to baby G, who loves playing with baby dolls?" Or "Let's give the Duplos to little Joshie since you are into Legos now." Be ready to take no for an answer. Often, they will give up something else instead. Or if it's a sentimental favorite, you can say, "Let's put these away for when you have kids," and put them into deep storage labeled "Grandkids."

Gear Bags

If your kid does activities like dance, sports, martial arts, or music, it helps to have all the gear for each activity stored in a separate backpack, tote, or duffle bag. That makes it easier to grab your gear bag and go on the day you have that activity. Just remember to take out the clothes or uniform to wash and put it back in the gear bag when they're clean. You might want hooks on the wall in their room for each gear bag, but some parents like to keep the bags by the front door (or closest to the car) so they don't forget them.

Memories, Schoolwork, and Artwork

A common concern for parents is what to do with the artwork, schoolwork, and memorabilia. I like to use under-bed storage containers for these things, which hold oversized items; even kids can pull them out and push them back easily. Pictures, letters, cards, invitations, programs, ticket stubs, and any physical evidence of happy memories also store well in an under-bed storage box.

You must check in with your kid to ensure you're saving only happy memories. Case in point: I was saving a trophy and uniform from my kid's season in Little League until he told me he was traumatized by the experience and didn't ever want to see those things again. Out they went!

Schoolwork can go in a second container. I keep reports, stories, projects, and journals. I also keep report cards, but in a file cabinet. For artwork, I keep the things made for holidays in that holiday storage container in the garage so I can see them every time I decorate for that holiday. I put everything else that's special and different in the under-bed container. I keep science project boards and odd-shaped things that don't fit in the container for a while and then take a picture and store that under the bed when I'm ready to get rid of the original. You can also take pictures of artwork that's either two-dimensional or three-dimensional and create a memory book in an app like Shutterfly. My daughter's 4th-grade teacher did that for each student, which was terrific.

If you try to keep everything, you will soon be overrun as your kids grow up. You've eventually got 18 years of stuff to save! I suggest going through the under-bed containers every summer with your kids. If they don't remember something or don't care if you get rid of it, consider whether you are ready to give it up. It's okay if you aren't; maybe you will be later when the containers are close to filling up.

12-Step Program for Cleaning Your Room

It took me years to realize that when I told my kids to clean their rooms, I didn't get compliance because they didn't know how. I developed this method with them, starting by making the bed. The room will look better already because at least one surface is clear. Then, everything on the floor gets picked up and put on the bed to sort and put away. This method works best when you have previously organized the room so everything has its place, although you may find more to declutter as you go. Even little kids can help pick up everything off the floor; a clear floor makes the room look neater.

By doing this daily or weekly with your kids, they will eventually learn to clean up this way, and it won't be so overwhelming. However, if your kids are neurodivergent (as mine are), they may not be able to do this without your help, even as they mature. You might want to leave these step-by-step directions inside their door with pictures to aid them.

1. Make your bed.
2. Pick up everything on the floor and the chairs and put it on the bed, except:
    a. Trash goes in the trash basket.
    b. Shoes go in the closet.
3. Deal with clothes:
    a. Is it dirty? If so, put it in the hamper.
    b. Does it fit? If it does, hang it up, fold it, and put it away.
    c. If it doesn't, put it in a pile outside the door to donate.
4. Now look for things that don't belong in the bedroom (dishes, silverware, and cups; someone else's stuff; stuff stored downstairs, etc.) and put them in the magic laundry basket.
5. Sort the rest by zone or area (closet, dresser, desk, bed, etc.)
6. Take everything for one zone and put it away, then do zone by zone until everything is off the bed.

7. Now go to each surface one by one (the top of the dresser, table, nightstand, desk) and repeat steps 3-6.
8. Dust with a Swiffer or wipe with a rag.
9. Sweep or vacuum.
10. Take out the trash and replace the bag.
11. Leave the laundry basket outside the room to take to another room
12. Bring the bag or box of donations to the front door.

Key Takeaway

It's easier for you and your kids to keep their rooms clean and organized if you set the room up with enough storage for each activity, and everyone knows where everything goes. Things should be stored in a way accessible for their height and easy to take out and put away so even young children can clean up by themselves.

PART 4

Handling Heavyweight Decisions

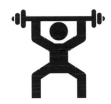

Chapter 18

Organize to Downsize

Now that you've established an organizing routine and built up those decision-making muscles, you're ready for some heavy lifting. At some point in your life, you will, most likely, encounter one of the most challenging organizing jobs: downsizing. Whether you are preparing for the future or have an immediate need, downsizing involves tough decisions, often based on available space.

The Most Stressful Events Include Moving

In 1967 the Holmes and Rhae Stress Scale was published, listing the most stressful events in our lives on a rating scale. I have consolidated the top ten into five: death of a loved one, change in marital status, imprisonment, personal injury or illness, and change of job status. What do all of those often have in common? Moving. Moving is stressful, even in the best of times, and if one of these other events makes it necessary to move, it is a double whammy. Planning a move is overwhelming for most people, even if they look forward to living in a new place, and it usually requires downsizing.

Decision-Making on Steroids

Downsizing is making decisions on steroids! Whether you are downsizing willingly or unwillingly, deciding what to eliminate when your world has been turned upside down is so stressful that many people pack everything and deal with it all later. Then you end up paying more to transport and store things for what could be months or years, only to dispose of them when you unpack.

Downsize Before You Move

Moving without downsizing first is why people have garages full of boxes, closets stuffed to the gills, and storage spaces they still pay for. When things settle down and you are in your "new normal," going through stuff you haven't missed is a low priority.

However, you will eventually have to go through things, and that looming prospect paralyzes people. But there comes a time when the stress of "I should" outweighs "I just can't." When that happens, it's time to open those boxes, go through the closets, empty those storage units, and reclaim your space and peace of mind.

Swedish Death Cleaning

To avoid all that extra work, why not downsize now, before you have to move? In Sweden, they call it Death Cleaning. You start downsizing your life now (meaning whole-home organizing) whether you are leaving your house or not, so your children don't have to do it when you die.

The Dreaded Garage

Ironically, I had just talked with my mom about downsizing while she was still young and healthy, and two weeks later, she was diagnosed with non-Hodgkin's lymphoma. A year later, she was gone without me having the chance to go through her home with her. Since my sister had been caring for my mom, she had to do most of it. Even in the best times, organizing is not my sister's forte. Distraught, my sister put off clearing the house until I could come up eight months later.

Cleaning the garage was the worst because my mom had run a childcare center out of her home and kept all kinds of recycled things most people would have considered garbage. But important papers, photos, and remnants of my childhood were mixed in, so I couldn't just chuck it all.

The kicker was when I found used wrapping paper from opened Christmas presents and tissue paper that I had used to wrap gifts for my friends' birthdays when I was in first grade. Fifty years later, that's what I wrapped my mom's stuff in when we packed it all up.

Please take my advice and don't leave it all for your kids to do.

Give It to Them Now

Go through your home with your adult kids or close family while you are well enough to do it. Tell stories, share memories, label pictures, and make it pleasant. If you are willing to part with something now, and your family tells you they want it, give it to them now to take home so they don't have to deal with it later when they are grief-stricken. Give your kids the remnants of their childhood: whatever is left of their room, school memories, and favorite toys saved for their kids.

If you're keeping something to pass down to your kids, ask them if they even want it. You'd be surprised at how many people are saving something that they think the kids will want and appreciate, and the kids have no interest, so it's been cluttering their home for years for no reason.

Suppose someone wants something they can't bring home yet. Label and document it so everyone knows. Write things of value into your will to protect siblings from fighting and future claims. Fights over their parents' things are one of the leading causes of estrangement among siblings.

If you don't have room to store their things because you are moving to a smaller place, consider whether it's worth renting a storage space to save it for them until they are settled.

Paring Down is Hard to Do

Downsizing is probably the toughest organizing challenge because the decisions are mainly based on available space.

My friend Dina was ruthless in downsizing when she and her husband went to live in a senior living community. She went from a two-story 4-bedroom house where she raised her kids to a 2-bedroom, one-level attached townhouse 45 years later.

She started at least a year ahead, paring down, room by room, closet by closet. Then when she leased the new place and knew its dimensions, she had to cut even more, taking just what was comfortable for her and her husband. She has never felt freer or happier in her whole life, and that's the best-case scenario.

Clutter-Blind

Downsizing is the hardest on people who have not built up a practice of decluttering and have never had to pack or pare down to fit a smaller space. Not only is there a lot of stuff, but the longer you live there, the less you see. Some people never notice their clutter unless it's in their way or they have to turn their house upside down to find something.

They become clutter-blind.

I had a client who lived in her house for 45 years and wanted to start "editing" now so she could move in a few years. Iris had become clutter-blind, and when we started working together, she discovered things she never knew she had. Conventional organizing wisdom says when you declutter, you should discard anything you don't use or love. But she wasn't ready to give up these things because she hadn't ever used them and now wanted a chance to enjoy them. It was like her home was one big department store full of new things she had paid for but forgot to bring home.

We spent more than a year decluttering one day a week, and during that time, she could enjoy the things she found, eventually getting rid of most of them.

You Don't Want to Be a Burden

If you haven't made a habit of organizing yet, I strongly suggest you start while you're healthy and before it's time to collect Social Security. I'm sure the last thing you want is to be a burden to anyone. Do I sound like a Jewish mother? Organize to help you downsize! And put on a sweater -- I'm cold.

Key Takeaway

Moving out is stressful enough, so you are doing yourself and your family a favor when you organize and downsize your home while you are still healthy before moving.

Chapter 19

Drowning in Paperwork

Paperwork should be called "paper-worst" because dealing with papers is usually the least enjoyable task of organizing your home. While going through piles of paper is tedious, the reward is a satisfying reduction of piles.

Paperwork is usually the last project to tackle. It helps to build up those decision-making muscles to do the heavy lifting of what to toss (or shred), what to save, where to file, and how long to keep.

The older you get, the worse it gets if you don't start a system now. The good news is that so much is online now. You don't have to keep actual papers if you are comfortable going online and getting what you need.

Paperwork is Paralyzing

I assisted a friend with organizing her home and business. Her husband was an accountant and naturally handled all their bills and finances. When he died suddenly, she could only take care of her child and clients. I handled all the paperwork and kept the lights on because she had never even seen an electricity bill, let alone paid one.

Handling her affairs was a full-time job. Because the husband's accounting firm was just him and a partner, there was no one to ask about life insurance, health insurance, and other personal accounts. I had to search his professional and home office to find important documents, including their marriage certificate, birth certificates, social security cards, insurance policies, titles to the cars, brokerage statements, open credit accounts, and the like.

That slowed down the process of applying for benefits and gaining access to liquid assets so they had money to live. I had to order death certificates and send them everywhere to close accounts and switch names.

The Green Binder

From that experience, I put together a 3-ring notebook (binder) with plastic page protectors containing all the essential documents in her life. I still encourage everyone to do the same. It works best when the binder is easily identifiable with a color not white or black, so you can tell someone, "It's all in the green binder in the file cabinet," or "look for the red binder at the bottom of the bookcase in my office."

This binder keeps all your important papers together in one place and makes it easy to have all the information you need when you are "taking care of business." You take it with you if you must evacuate and not miss a beat, even if you can never return home.

Taking time to put this binder together will reduce stress if you have to take on more paperwork than you usually do to keep things running.

Having the binder reduces the need to search for documents containing important information. It saves the worry that you might miss something, because if it is not contained or mentioned in the binder, you might not know that an account or document exists.

This binder will also be what the person managing your affairs needs if you become incapacitated or in the event of your passing. Tell your power of attorney (spouse, trustee, executor, fiduciary, adult children, trusted friend, or family member) where the binder is located so they can begin taking care of things immediately.

Information and Documents You Need

Think of all the information you need to fill out forms and have the authorization to access or close an account. That is the information you need for the binder.

Sometimes, you don't need the original document in the binder but at least a copy or a copy of the main page. For example, you only need a copy of your driver's license and the insurance policy declaration page; the rest of the insurance policy stays in a file folder.

For all your financial and online accounts, a page showing the account number, contact information, and online credentials (log-in and password) for access is enough. The rest you can leave in your files.

Update the information regularly, including your login and password for each account. Also include contact information for your spouse, children, family members, power of attorney, fiduciary, attorney, accountant, financial advisor, insurance agent, realtor, employer, and people who provide a service at your home.

Identity documents

- Birth certificate
- Passport
- Social security card
- Real ID or driver's license
- Military discharge papers
- Marriage certificate
- Dissolution of marriage certificate
- Legal name change
- Immigration status
- Work permit

Keep the original, make a copy, and have several official copies of certificates on hand to send out. If you are managing the estate of another, you will need to order at least a dozen death certificates so you can send them to entities that require them.

Legal documents that indicate your wishes

- Power of attorney
- Durable medical power of attorney
- Advance medical directive
- Will
- Trust documents
- Custody agreement
- Adoption or legal guardianship papers

Everything should be signed and dated (notarized if needed), and you should have the original and at least one hard copy. A trustee will probably need at least a dozen copies of power of attorney and certificate of trust documents.

Financial information

- Checking, savings, brokerage, and retirement account numbers and contact info
- Online login credentials for each account and financial institution
- Copy of debit card(s) (front and back) with PINs
- Blank check with the routing number for each account
- IRS payment plans
- Contact Information for the person who does your taxes and the location of the last seven years of tax returns
- Treasury account information (if you have bonds)
- Timeshare information (account number and location)

- Account numbers, billing information, and online credentials for all open credit accounts
  - Loans
  - Mortgages
  - Lines of credit
  - Credit cards

Insurance information

- Health
- Life
- Accidental Death and Dismemberment
- Disability
- Long Term Care
- Automobile
- Home
- Rental
- Earthquake
- General Liability
- Umbrella
- Pet

Include the name, account number, contact information, and online credentials for each account, plus the location of the policies and contact info for the insurance agent.

Vehicle Information (for each one you currently own)

- Lease or sale agreements
- Title and Registration
- Proof of Insurance and Declaration Page

Home documents for homes you currently own or rent

- Closing Escrow statement (copy)
- Mortgage statement (showing escrow account info if you have it)

- Property tax statement with assessed value
- Rental agreements with the property owner
- Renter contact information
- Title as currently written

Your trustee or executor will also need to know the appraisal value of each home at the time of death.

Government agencies from which you receive benefits

- Eligibility letter, account number, and login credentials for
  - Social Security
  - Medicare/Medicaid
  - Veterans Administration
  - Other social service programs
- Copy of EBT card and PIN.

Advance funeral arrangements

- Mortuary and cemetery contract and payment plan with plot number(s) and services (coffin, headstone, burial, cremation, urn, perpetual care, etc.)
- A list of funeral wishes to be honored.

Online Presence

Account name, login, and password for:

- Websites
- Email accounts
- Social media accounts
- Blogs
- Channels
- Subscriptions
- Streaming services
- ID monitoring services (i.e., LifeLock)

Medical and DNA Information

- List of current prescriptions and medical conditions
- Contact Information for primary care physicians, dentists, and specialists
- Cord blood bank information
- IVF embryo storage information
- Genetic testing company account number, login, and reports
- Fingerprints and DNA evidence for children's identification

What Else Do I Need to Save?

The Green Binder should also include a list of the following documents and whether they are located in physical files (hard copies in file folders) or digital files on your computer or cloud service where you can save and access files from any device (i.e., Google Drive, Apple iCloud, etc.).

It's important to know If you have a digital copy available so you don't go crazy looking for a hard copy, especially if you must email it to someone. Remember to include the username and password to access it. Here's another tip: if you can't find a digital copy you know exists, search your emails for those with attachments.

Taxes

- Tax Returns with documentation for the last seven years
    - W-2, 1099s
    - Interest statements
    - Receipts for deductions (donations, medical receipts, license fees)
    - Gas receipts if you get reimbursed
    - Log of miles driven for work (to write off)
    - Travel expenses (to write off)
- Tax Documentation for the year(s) you still need to file.

Home

- Homeowner or rental insurance policy
- Closing documents for homes you currently own
- Repair and remodeling receipts for homes you currently own
- Home warranty information (current year, if you have it)
- Property tax assessment documentation, if it has been adjusted
- Lease agreement
- Lease agreements for your tenants

Vehicles (only for vehicles you currently have)

- Auto insurance policy (all pages for the current year only)
- Repair receipts
- Finance agreement
- Lease agreement

Legal

- Divorce decree and current spousal support (alimony) agreement
- Custody and visitation agreement (until the last child is 18)
- Social security statements
- Public assistance records
- Trust documents and wills
- Trust documents, power of attorney, and death certificates if you are executor or trustee

Financial

- Mortgage and HELOC agreements (only current)
- Loan agreements (only current)
- Brokerage statements that show the price you paid for investments you hold
- Bank statements - 2 years (or online)
- Open credit card account agreements
- Bonds that haven't been entered online yet
- Time share agreements
- Monthly credit card statements unless you can get them online
- Print-out of year-end credit card statements downloaded into Excel
- Paid bills from this year and last year

Medical (by person)

- Current prescriptions and medical Info on fridge for EMT
- Prescription receipts or prescription history
- Test results
- Radiology reports (X-rays, CT scans, ultrasounds)
- Neuropsychological testing and reports

Warranties/Manuals

- Warranties and manuals with receipts attached, organized in files: Large Appliances, Small Appliances, Technology, Tools, Toys, Yard, etc.

School

- Report cards - throw out progress reports after the final grades arrive
- IEP, 504, and health plan documentation (including reports and testing)
- Standardized test results

Key Takeaway

Keep important documents and account information in a 3-ring binder, online folders, and physical file folders so you (or another designated person) can handle your affairs.

Chapter 20

You've Got Mail

Most of the piles of paper in your house come from the mail, and if you're like most of my clients, most of the mail you get can be thrown out immediately. When you pick up the mail, sort it at once. Rip up junk mail and throw it away. If you don't look at the grocery ads, newsletters, or catalogs, throw them out before they land anywhere. If you don't need a service someone sells (realtor, home improvement, insurance, etc.), toss it. Fundraising appeals from organizations you don't intend to support--gone. That's more than half of the mail you receive.

The rest of the mail goes into four piles: things to pay (bills), things to go to (invitations and appointments), things to take care of, and things to look at and then file.

Bills

You can save trees by getting billing statements online; however, if the charges change monthly and you do not look at your accounts online regularly, I recommend keeping the paper statements so you can keep an eye on your activity. I like to open the bills, throw away the envelope and extraneous pages, and put them in a file on my desk until I'm ready to pay them.

After I pay them, I store them in an expanding letter file by month, so I can look back if necessary. I keep two expanding files: this year's and last year's bills. At New Year's, this year's bills become last year's, and I trash or shred the contents of the year before to start the new year with an empty file. The assumption is you have done your taxes for that year. If you haven't, there are some bills you will want to save if you itemize medical or business deductions.

Invitations and Appointments

When I get an invitation or appointment confirmation, I schedule it in my Calendar app and then hang it on the fridge or a bulletin board or keep it on my desk so I see it in front of me. After the date has passed, I throw appointment papers out and put invitations in the memory box if I want to save them.

Things To Take Care Of

Things that need to be taken care of go in the inbox, and when you have completed the task, you can throw the paper away, put it in the pending file, or file it. For example, I get a notice in the mail about renewing my dog's license every year, and I pay online, then throw the paper away. When I get a renewal registration notice from the DMV, I pay online and put the notice in the pending file until the tags come. Then I put the DMV bill into the current year's Tax Receipts file so we can deduct the license fee on our tax return.

When I get a form in the mail, I fill it out, scan and attach it to an email, and then file it.

Things to Look at and File

Some things that come in the mail, like insurance policies and financial statements, only need to be reviewed and filed. Sometimes things like health insurance explanations of benefits are online, and you can opt not to get a hard copy sent in the mail. If you get hard copies, you can look at them and either file or throw them out, knowing you can get the information online if needed. That saves a lot of room in your file drawers.

"To File" Pile

I don't file everything immediately, and I don't expect you to, but I hope you create a filing system and put papers in a "to file" pile in an inbox-type container so that when you are ready to file, the papers have somewhere to go.

Reducing the Piles

Everybody has piles, and half the papers in them can probably be trashed. The trick is to take care of papers immediately when they enter your house so they don't become piles.

If you already have piles (and who doesn't?), you can manage them by following this sorting routine.

- Throw out the trash.
- Put the unpaid bills in a To Pay folder until they are paid.
- Put the paid bills in the expanding file by month except these (they are filed elsewhere):
  - Expenses to write off on your taxes
  - Expenses for home repairs
- Toss statements if they are the same amount each month (like mortgage or insurance) or if you can see them online
- File documents for tax returns in the current year's tax file
- Put things to take care of in the To-Do folder or inbox and schedule a time to take care of them!
- Put things you need to keep in the To File pile – but don't let it sit there for long! File a little each week so it doesn't overwhelm you.

Key Takeaway

Sort paperwork as soon as it comes into your home to minimize piles.

Chapter 21

It's Gotta Be Worth Something

Here are resources for appraising and selling online. The listing price of similar items can be helpful, but the final selling price is more important. Remember, something is only worth what a buyer will pay. If you have difficulty letting go, try selling online first; if things sell, great. If not, you can donate them and feel confident that at least you tried.

Appraisers

Value My Stuff Upload pictures of your item with any information you have. They assign an expert from their team of over 60 auction house specialists, and you receive an appraisal in 24-48 hours for less than $28. www.valuemystuff.com

Heritage Auctions This international auction house has an online appraisal form for potential auction material and offers formal written appraisals for estate planning and insurance. They also offer online value guides; you can search the archives to see how items sold in the past. www.ha.com

- Antiques & Art
- Autographs
- Books
- Coins and Currency
- Comics and Animation Art
- Home Entertainment and VHS
- Instruments and Vintage Guitars

- Jewelry
- Judaica
- Movie Posters and Memorabilia
- Music Memorabilia and Concert Posters
- Nature, Crystals, and Science
- Sports Memorabilia and Rare Sneakers
- Timepieces and Luxury Accessories
- Video Games, Trading Card Games, Action Figures, and Vintage Toys
- Wine

Baseball Cards www.psacard.com

Music (Vinyl, CDs, etc.) www.valueyourmusic.com

Sell In Person

Garage Sales and Flea Markets In my experience, garage sales are seldom worth the time and trouble for what little money you make, and you end up donating much of it anyway. If you have many things of value, you could get a booth at a flea market or swap meet where you may be required to pay a fee or commission, but you have a larger pool of motivated buyers. You still may bring home whatever doesn't sell or donate it anyway. Since many people don't carry cash, you can set up Venmo, PayPal, or Zelle to receive payments. No fee is involved if you are not a regular merchant and your account is attached to a bank account.

List Locally for Pickup or Ship

Facebook Marketplace, Craig's List, Offer Up

These online sites list your items for local pick-up (you can also offer to ship.) If you are uncomfortable having people come to your home, you can arrange to meet elsewhere. Arrange for payment at pickup (cash, Venmo, PayPal, Zelle), and don't fall for scams asking for something when they show interest in a listing.

- www.facebook.com/marketplace
- www.craigslist.com
- www.offerup.com

List Nationally and Ship Direct to Buyers

eBay: If you are willing to ship items and pay selling fees, eBay is a good choice for selling collectibles. The fees vary, so make sure it's worth your time and trouble to list and ship. You can get an idea of the value of something by watching auctions but remember: it's what people have paid, not what it's listed for, that counts.

www.ebay.com

Discogs: Sell individual vinyl records, CDs, cassettes, etc. No fee to list. When you sell an item, you are charged a flat fee of 8%, with a maximum fee of $150 per item.

www.discogs.com

Vinyl Record Network: Sell vinyl collections in lots of ten. The company takes a 25% commission on the selling price, and you ship straight to the buyer. A vinyl grading guide is available.

www.vinylrecordnetwork.com

Consignment

Estate Sales and Auctions: This online search tool finds estate sales and auction companies near you. They will appraise and price everything and take a percentage of the sales as a fee, which could be 20-40% for estate sales, depending on their services, and 10-30% for auctions. Some estate sale companies will also take things on consignment.

www.estatesales.net

Consignment Stores: If you have time to wait for a sale and are willing to pay a commission, consignment works well for designer clothing and accessories, quality children's clothing, and unique or like-new high-end furniture. Search online for stores near you, and call for what they accept and their commission.

The RealReal: This online authenticated luxury consignment shop takes 15%-40% commission. They accept women's, men's, and kids' fashion, fine jewelry and watches, home décor, and art. You can schedule a pickup, drop them off, or ship them. If you want to know what you can get for your Louis Vuitton, they have a handbag estimate tool to give you an idea of pricing.

www.realreal.com

Poshmark: This online retailer sells clothes, jewelry, home décor, electronics — pretty much anything. Sellers pay a flat commission of $2.95 for items under $15 and a 20% commission for items over $15. Shipping is easy; they email a label prepaid and pre-addressed. You package the item, print the label, and take it to USPS.

www.poshmark.com

Depop: This is a popular site for young fashionistas to turn their clothes into cash. Sellers list their clothes separately and ship them to buyers nationwide, and Depop emails a prepaid and pre-addressed label to print out. The seller's fee is 10% plus a PayPal or Depop transaction fee of about 3.5%.

www.depop.com

ThredUp: This online thrift store sends you a "clean up kit" to clean out your closet of gently used unwanted clothing and return the bag to them. Then they give you a payout depending on the price when the item sells. The higher the selling price, the higher percentage you get. ThredUp seems a no-brainer if you are not selling designer items, don't have time to manage listings and shipping, and plan to donate the clothes anyway

www.thredup.com

Chapter 22

Take My Stuff, Please

Donate

The Thrift Shopper: Visit this website and enter your zip code to find a list of thrift stores in your area that support your favorite cause. Contact the store first and ask if you can schedule a pickup, when you can drop off, and what, if anything, they are not accepting at the moment.

www.thethriftshopper.com

Habitat for Humanity ReStore: Habitat ReStores are home improvement stores that accept small and large donations of new or gently used furniture, appliances, housewares, building materials and more. Call first to make sure what they will accept.

www.habitat.org/restores

Retold Recycling for Textile Recycling: Retold sends bags for you to fill with 5 lbs. of donated clean, dry textiles in any condition to divert them from the landfill: clothes, blankets, towels, dishcloths, bed linen -- even old underwear, bras, cotton face masks, and rags! Each bag comes with a postage-paid label so you can drop it off at the post office - but the catch is you pay for shipping by buying a 10-pack of bags or a subscription of 6 bags a year. Saving the earth is not cheap!

www.retoldrecycling.com

Facebook Marketplace: List your item with $0 as the price, and buyers will contact you on Messenger. There are also Buy Nothing and similar Facebook groups to join that use the Marketplace format to offer items to their group members.

www.facebook.com/marketplace

Kars for Kids: You've probably heard the jingle. 1-877-Kars-4-Kids, donate your car today! Other groups (like veteran organizations) do the same, but this is the most visible car donation program. They take your vehicle, running or not, and you get a tax deduction.

www.kars4kids.org

Trash

Kick It to the Curb: In many areas, you can leave metal on the curb, and a metal collector makes it magically disappear by the morning. You can also try this for furniture because people often go "curb shopping."

Local Sanitation Department: Call to schedule a bulky item pickup for anything that doesn't fit in your garbage bin: broken appliances, used furniture, junk, or building materials. In some areas, you may be limited to only one or two pickups a year.

1-800-GotJunk: You pay for a pickup, but the advantage is that they take everything from wherever it is, so you don't have to carry it to the curb or wait until your next garbage day for a bulky item pickup. They supposedly donate what they can and take the rest to the dump. The price is based on how much space your junk takes up in the truck, and they tell you upfront when they arrive so you can take it or leave it. It may cost more than a hauling company. Call or go online to schedule. www.1800gotjunk.com

Hauling Company: They take everything to the dump for a fee: items you can't donate, junk, and debris. They are good to call when you are clearing out a house, and they are usually cheaper than 1-800-GotJunk because they are local businesses. Search online or ask for referrals.

Chapter 23

Size Does Matter

Sales of home organization products are expected to reach $13.5 billion in 2025. The Container Store alone does $895 million in business annually. Target, Walmart, Home Depot, Lowes, Costco, and Amazon carry a fantastic variety of containers online that you don't regularly find in the stores.

Whether using plastic, canvas, metal, wood, or cardboard containers, please ensure they are good quality products that will last. If it's something that you pull out all the time, it should be sturdy enough to withstand pulling and pushing without losing shape. Buy the right shape and size for the contents and location at whatever level of detail you feel is sufficient. For example, you can store basic art supplies in a shoebox from Target, but Michael's has specialized containers for crafters and artists to sort items to the n*th* degree.

Containers Should Fit the Shelves

Look for containers made explicitly for the depth of closet and cabinet shelves and can stack. Big containers should fit two or three across on steel shelving, and containers with straight walls fit better side by side. If you have a choice between a huge container or two smaller ones, consider how much you can carry. If you need help to lift a container up and down, you are less likely to put things away, and clutter will accumulate.

Before you shop, measure all your shelves' width, depth, and height. Be aware of irregularities: you may not be able to go to the edge of a shelf if the door needs space to close. Or you may have to adjust the height measurement if you lift a container over a lip on the shelf instead of simply sliding it in.

If your shelves are not adjustable, make sure the containers with their lids on will fit under the shelf above them. You can maximize your space by buying the right size containers to fit two or three across a shelf without too much space left over.

If you're not using containers on the shelves, shelf dividers are great for keeping stacks of clothes, towels, sheets, and handbags neat on shelves.

Typical Shelf Depths

Kitchen

- Upper cabinet shelf: 10.5"D
- Lower cabinet shelf: 19.25"D
- Under Sink: 22.5"D
- Pantry shelf: 20"D
- Pantry drawer: 19.5"D

Hall Closet

- Top Shelf: 16.5"D
- Floor: 27"D

Linen Closet

- Deep Shelf: 22"D
- Shallow Shelf: 14"D

Laundry Room

- Cabinet shelf: 12"D or 15"D

Bathroom Cabinet

- Regular under sink: 19.5"D
- Powder room under sink: 11.5"D

Bedroom Closet

- Wire shelf: 12"D
- Closet system shelf: 14"D
- Floor: 27"D

Bookcases

- Shelves: 11"-12"D x 10"-13"H
- Cubbies for fabric cubes: 11"W x 13"H x 15"D or 13"W x 11"H x"14" D (depending on orientation)

Steel Shelving

- Gorilla Rack: 24"D
- Wire Rack on Casters: 14"D
- Baker's Rack: 14"-18"D

Storage Ideas

The best way to store anything is the way that works best for the person who is putting things away. Here are some methods:

Shoes:

- 6 qt shoe box
- Paired on a shelf at least 10.5"D

Boots:

- 12 qt box
- boot hangers if you have hanging space

Hats:

- Hatbox for big hats
- Cap hanger

Pants:

- Folded in thirds on shelves, retail style
- Folded on hanger
- Hung long on clips (skirt hanger)

T-shirts

- Folded on shelves, retail style
- Hung
- Rolled in drawers

Sweatshirts

- Folded on shelves, retail style
- Hung

Towels

- Folded in thirds or halves, with the fold facing out
- Folded in thirds and rolled in a basket, cubby, or shelf

Sheets

- Folded with sets stored together or inside the pillowcase on a shelf

Handbags

- On shelves like books

Seasonal clothes and accessories

- In containers on a closet shelf

Memories

- Underbed Containers, ideally with wheels and a split top

Depending on your bed frame, you can store one under a twin, two under a full or queen, and up to four under a king.

Chapter 24

Before and After

So there you have it. All the wisdom I have to send you on your organizing journey, except one little secret I forgot to mention:

It always looks worse before it gets better.

Don't be discouraged when you see yourself surrounded by everything you pulled out or piles sorted on the floor. It's easy to lose motivation when the mess inside is now on the outside. But it's only temporary! It's part of the process, so I advise you to only pull out one shelf, cabinet, or drawer at a time.

Practice organizing the easy rooms – kitchen, bathrooms, and common rooms – first. Then move on to the occupied bedrooms with the help of the people who sleep there. Only then can you move on to the heavyweight division – the dreaded garage, the basement, and the rooms that aren't used daily, the ones you can close the door to and try to forget they exist.

You can do this! You now have the tools and the strength to continue organizing because you can look at things, feel the emotions as they arise, and make decluttering decisions based on "Is this good for me?"

Maintaining an organized home is maintaining your mental health, confidence, and self-esteem. Creating a peaceful environment where you can relax is one of the best gifts you can give to yourself, and being able to invite people into your home proudly is priceless.

I recently discovered a Facebook page for declutterers where people post their "before" and "after" pictures to show their accomplishments. When I start a new organizing job with a client, I usually dive in and forget to take pictures.

Still, I encourage you to do it because once you start decluttering and organizing, the transformation will feel so natural that you will forget how it used to look. I want you to see your progress and love the "after" in your home and yourself.

If you get stuck, need encouragement, or want to show off your accomplishments, I am always a call, email, Facebook page, or Google Meet away. And remember my mantras:

- You don't have to do it all at once; you just have to do it.
- Keep the best and reduce the rest.
- Practice makes progress, not perfection.

And last but not least:

Done is better than perfect!

End Notes

[1]Vartanian, L. R., Kernan, K. M., & Wansink, B. (2017). Clutter, chaos, and overconsumption: The role of mind-set in stressful and chaotic food environments. *Environment and Behavior, 49*(2), 215-223. doi:10.1177/0013916516628178

[2]Cutting, J. E., & Armstrong, K. L. (2016). Facial expression, size, and clutter: Inferences from movie structure to emotion judgments and back. *Attention, Perception, & Psychophysics, 78*(3), 891-901. doi:10.3758/s13414-015-1003-5

[3]Amer, T., Campbell, K. L., & Hasher, L. (2016). Cognitive control as a double-edged sword. *Trends In Cognitive Sciences, 20*(12), 905-915. doi:10.1016/j.tics.2016.10.002

[4]Lucassen PJ, Pruessner J, Sousa N, Almeida OF, Van Dam AM, Rajkowska G, Swaab DF, Czéh B. Neuropathology of stress. Acta Neuropathol. 2014 Jan;127(1):109-35. doi: 10.1007/s00401-013-1223-5. Epub 2013 Dec 8. PMID: 24318124; PMCID: PMC3889685.

[5]Justin B. Echouffo-Tcheugui, Sarah C. Conner, Jayandra J. Himali, Pauline Maillard, Charles S. DeCarli, Alexa S. Beiser, Ramachandran S. Vasan, Sudha Seshadri.Circulating cortisol and cognitive and structural brain measures. Neurology Nov 2018, 91 (21) e1961-e1970; DOI: 10.1212/WNL.0000000000006549

About the Author

Donna Barwald owns Neatly Arranged Professional Organizing in Los Angeles, organizing homes, offices, and special events. She also consults virtually. A Jewish mother and recovering perfectionist, Donna gives practical advice about organizing challenges and decluttering dilemmas. Between projects, Donna can be found on her sofa binge-watching anything with subtitles and cuddling with her cat.

Email: NeatlyArrangedOrganizing@gmail.com
Website: www.neatlyarranged.com
Blog: neatlyarranged.substack.com
Facebook: facebook.com/NeatlyArrangedOrg